# "LET ME TELL YOU SOMETHING, DR. WILSON"

## What I Learned From My Patients

Dr. Jeffrey W. Wilson

*"Let Me Tell You Something, Dr. Wilson"*
*What I Learned From My Patients*

© 2016

Dr. Jeffrey W. Wilson

ISBN: 978-0-9978020-4-7

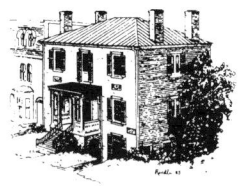

Warwick House Publishers
720 Court Street
Lynchburg, Virginia 24504

*Dedicated to Sandra, Elizabeth, and Melissa.*
*Thank you for tolerating my mistress over forty years.*

"Live a simple and a temperate life,
that you may give all your powers to your profession.
Medicine is a jealous mistress;
she will be satisfied with no less."
—Sir William Osler

"Duke is not for everybody,
and medicine is a demanding mistress."
—Eugene A. Stead, Jr., M.D.

# CONTENTS

# INTRODUCTION

## "THAT'S NOT DISCOMFORT, THAT'S PAIN!"

It must have been at least the twentieth time I had inject-ed one of Jean's joints in the last three years, and she'd had enough—at least enough of my usual spiel. After prepping the joint with betadine, I would spray on topical skin refrigerant to decrease the pain of injection and just before the needle hit the skin, I would say, "Jean, there's going to be a little discomfort." Imagine hearing that line twenty times followed by a painful injection. You would have the same response, "Let me tell you something, Dr. Wilson, that's not discomfort, that's pain!" After that, as I was about to inject a joint, I'd say, "Jean, there's going to be a little (long pause) pain." We would both laugh, but only after the injection was finished.

Jean's good-natured critique not only provided a lesson about discomfort versus pain, but was an example of the many things patients told and taught me over the past thirty-five years. One definition of "doctor" is "teacher." Indeed, most physicians in non-surgical specialties spend the majority of time teaching their patient about illness, health risk factors, and treatments. Sometimes, however, we need to be the student and learn by listening to the patient.

But the doctor as "listener" is an endangered species now as office visits are shortened and the physician has parameters of documentation that must be met to satisfy coding require-ments for Medicare and insurance reimbursement. Documenta-tion in this era of the electronic medical record (EMR) trumps listening.

A common complaint by patients now is decreased per-sonal interaction when the doctor comes in the exam room with a laptop computer. The physician may not even look at the patient as data is entered into the EMR from a directed interview. One patient said the doctor never touched her for a physical exam, only typing on the laptop. So much for the healing touch, and I bet we never hear a patient complain that the doctor spent too much time listening to them.

The drawing below was displayed on a wall in my office. It was made by a Navy officer in 1976 as appreciation for taking

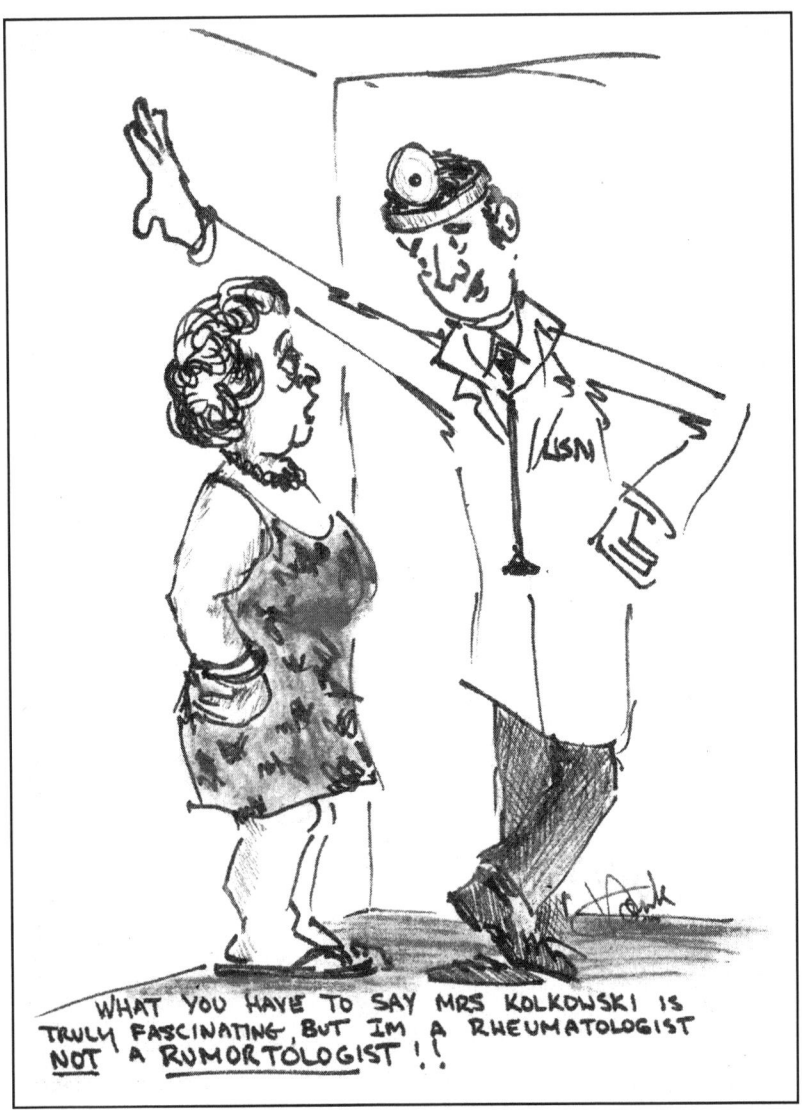

WHAT YOU HAVE TO SAY MRS KOLKOWSKI IS TRULY FASCINATING, BUT IM A RHEUMATOLOGIST NOT A RUMORTOLOGIST !!

care of his daughter's juvenile arthritis. It depicts a caricature of me as a young Navy doctor explaining to a portly female patient, "What you have to say, Mrs. Kolkowski, is truly fascinating, but I'm a rheumatologist, not a rumortologist." Little did I suspect that over the next thirty-five years I would be both.

Perhaps it relates to the nature of arthritis ills or the rheumatologist-patient relationship, but patients have always shared stories and advice, as Jean did, related to diagnosis and treatment of their conditions. One day as a patient outlined a litany of unconventional treatments including garlic, gin-soaked raisins and DMSO, I finally interrupted and asked what her primary care physician thought about all of this. "Oh, I would never tell *him* something like this," she replied. My immediate thought was, "Why *me*, then?"

And I would have been wrong. While the physician needs to know about alternative, complementary, over-the-counter therapies, or home remedies, more importantly taking time to listen to the patient's stories will advise and educate us. We gain an insight into the unique personality of our patient. It helps us become more effective physicians, maybe even "rumortologists." Listening enriches the practice and the art of medicine.

In the following pages let me share with you things my patients told and taught me. Some stories are funny, humbling, or sad, but hopefully all are informative and interesting. With over thirty-five years of practice in Lynchburg, most of this education has come from my Central Virginia patients. I thank them.

Jeffrey W. Wilson, M.D
January 4, 2016


Note: HIPAA (Health Insurance Portability and Accountability Act) prohibits identifying any patient directly, and the narratives that follow, while based on actual patient encounters, have names changed unless specifically permitted by the patient or family members.

# "YOU DIDN'T KNOW WHAT YOU WAS DOING, DID YOU?!"

## (Lupus)

Sometimes the education is humbling. I had taken care of Samantha (Sam) for several years since starting my Lynchburg rheumatology practice in July 1979. She was an African American high school student struggling with lupus. In spite of recurrent flares with skin rash, mouth sores, chest pain, and arthritis, she had a sparkling personality, remained active in E. C. Glass singing groups, and was described once by her teachers as a "shining penny."

At that time, a commercial medical laboratory provided free lab tests for indigent patients if the doctor did not charge the patient. This worked well because labs to follow the course of lupus often involve expensive tests such as complement levels, anti-DNA, and other antibody tests much more costly than our routine urinalysis, sed rate (sedimentation rate), or CBC (complete blood count). She was followed at no charge in our office with this valuable benefit of free lab tests. Sometimes, however, in spite of maintenance therapy with prednisone and Plaquenil (hydroxychloroquine), Sam would have to be admitted to the hospital. On one occasion, she had a systemic infection and I admitted her for intravenous antibiotics.

From the time I started practice, under the advice of a mentoring physician, the late Dr. Wilbur Burger, I took Wednesday afternoon and evening off each week. Some patients thought there was an unspoken rule allowing only half the doctors to work on Wednesday and the other half working on Thursday— all doctors golfing on one day or the other. As a non-golfer, I can assure you this is not so; some of us are fishing.

In any event, during this particular hospitalization, on Wednesday night, the nurse and IV team could not keep an

IV going for her antibiotics. The paging service directed the call from 3D floor at LGH (Lynchburg General Hospital) to my home number instead of to the on-call physician. I thought it must be providential. Somehow, I was meant to be called—but I was worried. As a medical student and house officer (intern and resident), I drew all the blood for tests and started my own IVs. I became proficient and felt I could draw blood from a stone and start an IV on anyone. But that had been several years earlier and I had since learned that when neither the nurse nor the IV team could maintain or start an IV, I was unlikely to succeed in finding venous access. However, feeling a special obligation, I headed back to the hospital around 9:00 PM. Anticipating problems, I asked the nurses to wrap Sam's arms in warm-wet soaks, a trick learned during house staff training days to make the veins more prominent and easier to find when starting an IV.

As I drove to the hospital, I felt a sense of pride. My med school professors would surely approve answering the call to come to the aid of a patient on my night off, an example of care that money can't buy. The story should end with the successful placement of an IV, assuring access for the antibiotics. But, no. For over two hours, we soaked Sam's arms, patted hands and forearms to get the veins to stand up, and poked and prodded with multiple IV catheters—to no avail. After nine sticks and no success, Sam and I both raised the white flag of surrender. Sam was sweating from fear and pain, and I was a sweaty mess from frustration and failure. We would have to settle for intramuscular shots of antibiotics. The ride home was one of deflated pride and ego. Perhaps my old Duke professors would be more amused than proud.

The next day as I made rounds, Sam still had warm-wet soaks ministering to her now bruised and punctured arms. She looked up as I entered her room and said, "Dr. Wilson, you know last night when you came in here…" (Frankly, I was surprised. Only seventeen years old but apparently she understood and was going to acknowledge and thank me for this special care and attention.) Instead, Sam continued, "…you didn't know what you was doing, did you?!" Stunned and shocked,

5

but mainly humbled, I responded, "Sam, you're right. And the next time you need help in the middle of the night, don't let the nurses call me. Call someone who knows what they're doing!"

# "I'M NOT PAYING FOR THIS VISIT"
## (The Problem of Pain)

The patient stormed out of the office with this parting message. I had spent the majority of the appointment time trying to explain that pain meds were not the way to treat his rheumatoid arthritis, that there is a difference between pain and inflammation. This had been impressed upon me over forty years earlier during medical school and house staff training. A patient followed in the diabetic clinic would come in and ask to have his foot checked. "It doesn't hurt, but it doesn't work right." It was hard to believe that the swollen, deformed foot wasn't horribly painful. X-rays showed destructive changes in foot and ankle bones. The patient had a Charcot foot. As a consequence of his diabetes, the patient had lost pain sensation in the foot. Without the protective effect of pain, the foot quickly underwent marked destructive changes. Pain was a protector, not the problem. Other rarer conditions such as syringomyelia, leprosy, and congenital indifference to pain show similar phenomena of destroyed joints in the absence of pain. A book, *The Gift of Pain*, by Philip Yancey and Dr. Paul Brand, expounds in further detail on the protective effect of pain, beginning with Dr. Brand's experience caring for leprosy patients.

Pain is one manifestation of inflammation. Rubor (redness), tumor (swelling), calor (heat), and dolor (pain) are the classic features of inflammation. Patients with an inflammatory condition like rheumatoid arthritis need to primarily have the inflammation controlled. It is inflammation that can cause destruction of the joint, and pain may be a protective mechanism. It won't allow the patient to overuse and damage the inflamed joint. As I pointed out to my patient, if we control the inflammation, we protect the joint and decrease the pain. But this patient was not there to be educated; he was there for his pain meds—his Lortabs (hydrocodone).

Pain is a special problem. It is the most common reason a patient comes to see a doctor. Over fifteen years ago, a worrisome movement developed. It was based on the idea that no one should suffer any pain. Strong meds including opioid narcotics should be used to minimize or eliminate pain. The proponents contended that chronic use of these medications could be handled without severe addiction problems. Many physicians, myself included, remained skeptical. The grading of pain on a 0 to 10 scale became popular. Signs in the ER encouraged patients to let the doctor know if their pain was not relieved. It occurred to me that an addict would discover Nirvana, subjectively grading his pain at high levels to have more or stronger meds administered. Over the next few years, we began to see a proliferation of legitimate pain clinics and pain specialists, but also fraudulent opportunistic oxycontin clinics where the doctor would see over fifty patients a day and simply fill out prescriptions without examining the patient. I suspect that many urgent care clinics became a bonanza for patients seeking Lortabs, Percocet, or similar meds.

It came as no surprise that these strong medicines *did* result in abuse and addiction. Statistics for the last few years show over 380,000 ER visits a year are related to narcotic abuse and more than 20,000 deaths are attributed to these meds (since 2008 opioid analgesic overdose has caused more fatalities than motor vehicle accidents). *Prescribed* narcotics were the number one cause of ER visits and deaths from drug overdose—not illicit drugs like heroin or cocaine (*New England Journal of Medicine,* May 29, 2014 "Medication-assisted Therapies—Tackling the Opioid-Overdose Epidemic." Volkow, N. D. et al., p 2063).

Maybe if Adam and Eve had not messed up in the Garden of Eden there would be no pain. But they did, and we will all experience pain. While there are legitimate chronic pain patients who need the availability of all modalities for pain relief, we need to be cautious in the general use of these meds. Pain may be a warning that something is wrong, but it may also have a protective effect, especially in our arthritis patients by not allowing them to overuse and destroy an inflamed joint.

The government is taking steps to control the abuse of prescription opioids. On March 15, 2016, the Centers for Disease Control and Prevention (CDC) released a set of guidelines for prescribing opioids and the FDA wants to see training courses for physicians. Anyone who has dealt with drug or other forms of addiction in family members knows how difficult the problem can be. I would hope that education of the public, as well as physicians, is a priority. Otherwise, I suspect we'll see a shift of overdose and abuse problems from prescribed opioids to heroin and other street drugs. Time will tell.

Addendum: Since the time this essay was written in April, there is evidence that a shift to illicit drugs is already occurring. In June 2016, the Virginia State Office of the Chief Medical Examiner reported an increase in the number of severe overdose reactions to heroin often mixed with fentanyl [a black market drug 80 to 100 times stronger than heroin, manufactured by labs in Mexico and South America]. The same problem was reported in July 2016, by Massachusetts General Hospital ER in a letter to the editor *New England Journal of Medicine*.

# "I CAN'T BELIEVE YOU'RE GOING INTO RHEUMATOLOGY"

The morning of July 1, 1977, marked the beginning of sub-specialty training in rheumatology and my friend, Dr. Jeff Crawford, stunned me with his comment. He elaborated, "It's such a depressing field. How can you stand to take care of those arthritis patients? They're all a bunch of whiny passive dependents."

Normally, I would not pay any attention to such a remark but, on that same day, Dr. Crawford was starting his fellowship in hematology-oncology. When the cancer doctor thinks your field is depressing, maybe it's time for some introspection. How *did* this happen?

One of the godfathers of medicine, Sir William Osler, past chairman of the Department of Medicine at Johns Hopkins (1889-1905), suggested that when the arthritis patient came in the front door of the office, the appropriate response by the doctor was to go out the back door! Authoritative textbooks of rheumatology devoted entire chapters to the "rheumatoid personality," the patient portrayed as a chronic complaining, passive dependent individual unable to be helped. If you believed this, then my oncology friend was right.

I knew nothing about rheumatology until my final year of medical school. A classmate took the clinical elective and recommended the rotation mainly because the staff members were fun to work with, the rotation was easy, not too time consuming, and they had a beer party every Friday afternoon. While all this was true, I found this subspecialty of medicine to be fascinating. Impressive members of the rheumatology division began my education in the art and science of medicine, which would influence my practice forever: the importance of touch when seeing the patient and the uniqueness of the rheumatologist's joint exam and handshake (*never* a firm, painful grip). The patience in dealing with chronic disease processes, analyzing

10

clinical situations and planning treatment strategies for years to come are special to the rheumatology field and patient.

During medical school and internal medicine training, we are attuned to the acute disease processes with more attention to failing heart, lungs, or kidneys. It is exciting to give intravenous medications to diurese the heart failure patient or control arrhythmias. Urgent treatments often produce rapid, dramatic results. While concentrating on these acute illnesses, it's not unusual for the medical student to complete training with little knowledge about arthritis or the musculoskeletal exam. The rheumatology field seemed unique and there was special excitement as this was the first internal medicine subspecialty to bond with new developments in immunology. But it was the patients I encountered who influenced my choice of rheumatology as a career.

H. F. was fifty-five years old when I first met him during my student elective rheumatology rotation. He was afflicted with a complicated combination of rheumatoid and psoriatic arthritis. Marked crippling changes in his hands left him with completely useless fingers. This especially severe form of psoriatic arthritis is appropriately called arthritis mutilans. The rheumatoid component was likewise complicated with extra-articular (outside the joint) features including nodules, skin sores, anemia, low white blood cell counts, an enlarged spleen (Felty's Syndrome), and fluid around lungs (pleural effusions) and heart (pericardial effusion). Amazingly, he had continued physically demanding work as a butcher for seven years with active, progressive arthritis resistant to treatment. He was now totally disabled, unable to manage the activities of daily living such as feeding or cleaning himself. In this frail condition he faced the difficult decision of chest surgery without self-pity or fear. He was strengthened by his faith and a marvelous supportive wife and daughter who kept him involved and relevant in all aspects of the family life. He made final decisions regarding his medical or surgical treatment.

H. F. and his family taught me that our mind and spirit make us unique, not our physical bodies. The operation to strip

11

the sack from around the heart (pericardiectomy) was successful and H. F. was discharged.

Our paths crossed again the next year when I was the intern assigned to the rheumatology service. H. F. was losing weight, going from 165 lbs. down to 103 lbs., and had persistent infections. There was a chronic draining chest tube on his right side and he had multiple skin sores and ulcers. These were manifestations of Felty's Syndrome progressing to the point that another surgery, a splenectomy, was indicated. In his state of inanition, this surgery was riskier than last year's pericardiectomy. Another decision bravely faced. At surgery, he was found to have a spleen the size of a football. Post-operative convalescence was complicated by a heart attack.

Making rounds late one night, I stopped at H. F.'s room. Internship hours were traditionally long; you were on call five nights out of seven and you were always tired. After checking for any chest pain and examining heart and lungs, I reassured him that everything was stable. As I headed out the door, H. F. called to me, "Hey, Doc, I hope you get home tonight. You look tired and the family and I are worried you might be working too hard." Let's see. Post-op, terrible arthritis, recent heart attack, and H. F. and his family were concerned about me. No whiny, passive dependent patient here.

It was patients like H. F. whose courage, sensitivity, and unique personalities influenced me to choose rheumatology. I have no regrets. Most rheumatology patients show a similar magnificent spirit in dealing with the chronic challenges of serious inflammatory diseases like rheumatoid arthritis and lupus. These illnesses are not for the faint-hearted.

Two years of military service in the Navy (1974-1976) provided another perspective on medical care. During internship and residency, I practiced acute care when assigned to rotations on the cardiac care unit, respiratory care unit, medical intensive care unit and the emergency room. Like my fellow house officers (interns and residents), I enjoyed the dramatic medical care delivered. But when I returned to Duke in 1976, I noticed that few of the severe cardiac or pulmonary disease patients were still around. However, I often encountered former rheumatology patients. It affirmed my decision to become a rheumatologist. I would have the opportunity to make treatment decisions that could benefit patients for years to come. That always remained a great attraction of the subspecialty for me.

So, while Dr. Crawford could not believe I was going into rheumatology, I can't imagine doing anything else. It has been a privilege and honor to care for these patients.

# "I'M NOT TAKING THAT DAMNED CANCER MEDICINE"

## (Methotrexate)

Dr. Robert Bowden is a personal friend and fellow physician. More than twenty-five years ago, he was afflicted with a double dose of inflammatory arthritis: a combination of rheumatoid arthritis (RA) and spondyloarthropathy. Standard therapies, including a course of gold shots, were ineffective. Daily doses of 20 to 40 mg of prednisone were barely sufficient to keep him functioning. Bob was one of our finest OB-GYN physicians. He was at the peak of his career, his three sons were college age, and we worried if he would be able to continue his current practice. We even considered a psychiatry residency—training for a less physically demanding profession.

Out of desperation, for over twelve weeks we met each Wednesday as my morning clinic ended. I drained fluid from both knees and injected them with cortisone. The dictum from our orthopedic friends advised that a large joint like the knee could only be injected two or three times a year without destroying the joint. I warned Bob, "You'll probably need joint replacements after all these injections." His response? "If I don't get the injections I can't practice."

We were clinically between a rock and a hard place. Bob and I are "Old School" doctors. We like taking care of patients and the thought of going on disability, while ending practice, was an untenable option. The risks of steroid side effects and joint replacements were acceptable to continue practice as long as possible.

At that time, methotrexate was just being introduced as a new medicine for arthritis. Prior to this, methotrexate was in the oncologist's province as a chemotherapy agent. Bob's response foreshadowed a sentiment I would hear for the rest of my practice life. "I'm not taking that damned cancer medicine!"

I explained that we don't use methotrexate as a chemotherapy agent. When the rheumatology investigators at the NIH (National Institutes of Health) approached the oncologists about trying this new medicine for rheumatoid arthritis, the proposed initial dose of 7.5 mg weekly seemed laughable to the cancer doctors. That small dose could not possibly be effective. In rheumatology, however, we are not trying to mimic the effects of chemotherapy. Our smaller doses act as a DMARD (Disease Modifying Anti-Rheumatic Drug) with much less toxicity or side effects. We look for an immunomodulatory effect. That is, we don't want to suppress the immune system so severely that it can't perform its function fighting infection, but we do want to control its over-reaction against the patient's own body (the nature of autoimmune diseases like RA and lupus).

With gold therapy, we worried more about kidney function than bone marrow or liver toxicity. Methotrexate was a good alternative with more attention to liver toxicity than bone marrow or kidney side effects. However, with more concern for liver function, it was recommended that the patient abstain from alcohol and have a liver biopsy every two years with frequent blood tests monitoring for any methotrexate toxicity.

Doctors make interesting patients. We all have what I call the "Christmas effect" of medicine. We would rather give than receive medical care. Remember, most of us went through our medical education imagining we had the illnesses we were studying in pathology or observing on clinical rotations. Some of us are embarrassed to be sick. Is the illness seen as a sign of weakness? One physician I cared for insisted on coming in when no patients were in the office. Bob was exactly the opposite, charming my patients as he conversed with them in the waiting room. His practice probably increased as a result. However, he let me know that he would have his glass of wine each night and was not about to have a liver biopsy! So much for the compliant patient.

Over the next two years, Bob's arthritis went into remission. The frequent monitoring of blood tests showed no liver intolerance to methotrexate or wine, and by the time a liver biopsy would have been recommended, national experience following this new arthritis medicine suggested we did not need routine liver biopsies. "I told you so," was Bob's response to the news.

Prednisone was discontinued and gradually we began to taper the methotrexate. When the dose was down to one tablet weekly, and seeing no evidence of active arthritis, I delivered the good news, "Bob, you're in remission, you can stop the methotrexate."

"No way. I'm never stopping that medicine," he responded.

"You mean that damned cancer medicine you weren't going to take?" I asked.

"Exactly."

Bob eventually came off methotrexate, his arthritis remained in remission, and he completed his private practice OB-GYN career and still works at the Free Clinic in Lynchburg and Virginia Beach. He never needed knee replacements after the series of weekly injections. The rule of no more than two or three injections a year may apply to the osteoarthritic knee, but when active inflammation is present, there is probably significant protective effect achieved by removing inflammatory fluid and injecting cortisone.

# "I CAN'T BELIEVE YOU'RE MOVING TO THAT STAGNANT LITTLE VIRGINIA TOWN"

This was my mother-in-law's reaction when we announced our intention to begin practice in Lynchburg. She may have had an ulterior motive. She and my father-in-law hoped we might end up in their home town of Charlotte. But Sandra and I made the decision to practice in Lynchburg a full year before I finished my rheumatology fellowship in July 1979. Prior to med school (1968-1972), the only thing I knew about the city was via a fraternity brother from Lynchburg. Carl Patterson of the Patterson Pharmacy family was a fellow Sigma Nu. We made a cursory trip through Lynchburg on a fraternity pledge visit to see "the rock of Sigma Nu" at VMI where the fraternity was founded. I don't recall any outstanding impression. It seemed like a nice, quiet Virginia town.

It was later that Sandra and I began to discover Lynchburg when looking for the closest access to the Appalachian Trail (AT) from Durham. On an occasional day off during medical school, we would drive our two Dodge Darts up 501 N toward the AT access above Big Island. Leaving one car along the road where the trail comes down to 501 (now near the James River Foot Bridge), we would drive the other car north, parking at the trail intercept on the Blue Ridge Parkway. The eight or nine mile hike began with an ascent of Bluff Mountain to a fire tower (since burned down), followed along the ridge, and then wound down toward the James River trail end. Gathering both Dodge Darts, we would stop for supper at the Steer Barn Restaurant before driving back to Durham. After a day hiking outdoors, we were famished and I don't remember a salad bar, soup tureen and steak ever tasting better.

As we traveled through Lynchburg on 501, we were impressed with E. C. Glass High School—larger than some colleges in my home state of West Virginia. We drove by lovely homes along Langhorne Road. Hiking trips became less frequent after med school graduation (1972) and beginning post-graduate training in internal medicine. After our first child, Elizabeth, was born September 2, 1973, Lynchburg remained a nice memory, but infrequent destination.

Internal medicine training was interrupted with a two-year sojourn in the Navy. Returning to Duke in 1976 with our second child, Melissa, I began a senior residency year in internal medicine before starting a rheumatology fellowship in 1977. We considered practices in Raleigh, Greenville/Spartanburg area, Wilmington and Charlotte, North Carolina. Published practice guidelines suggested that a population of 200,000 was necessary to support a rheumatologist. We decided Lynchburg was a nice city, but too small (around 70,000) for a rheumatologist. Then, providence and Dr. Wilbur Burger entered our lives.

One of my friends completing a fellowship in Hematology/Oncology was being recruited by Wilbur and his partner, Dr. John Halpin, for the nascent Lynchburg Hematology and Oncology Clinic. Wilbur was a pioneer in bringing subspecialty medicine to Lynchburg. He started out practicing internal medicine with special interest in hematology/oncology as part of Dr. Charles Sackett's group. Realizing that he wanted to pursue the more subspecialized practice, Wilbur built a separate office and began his clinic. The practice with John was growing rapidly, and they were eager to recruit another physician.

In post graduate medical training, we maintained an informal network of communication among fellows in different specialties— interested in possible practice opportunities. Without Facebook or I-phones, we knew where our peers were being recruited. Hearing that one of the hematology/oncology fellows was looking at Lynchburg, the most casual inquiry changed everything. "Ask if they need a rheumatologist." Wilbur called immediately. With nothing to gain in terms of his own practice needs, he really recruited us to Lynchburg.

For the next year, I received a call every two to three weeks from Wilbur. Wilbur and his wife, Libby, hosted a visit to Lynchburg, which included a trip to Smith Mountain Lake, a great meal at Emil's Restaurant and interviews with physicians in town. Orthopedists, Paul Fitzgerald, Davis Von Oesen and Jay Hopkins were encouraging, Jay stating that Lynchburg was "ripe" for a rheumatologist. Of special importance, in our consideration, was an introduction to Dr. William Massie. Bill had one year of rheumatology training at the University of Virginia and practiced primarily internal medicine. In contrast to a Roanoke rheumatologist who saw no need for another rheumatologist (or competition) in his area, Bill encouraged us to come to Lynchburg. His patients loved him, he practiced excellent rheumatology and he was certainly not threatened by another rheumatologist. The visit with Bill and his wife, Annie Robertson Massie, introduced us to the epitome of Virginia southern charm and courtesy. Sandra and I will always be indebted to the Burgers and Massies for influencing our decision to live and practice in Lynchburg.

Once the decision was made to set up practice in Lynchburg, Wilbur's help continued. Calls regarding office space, recommendation for a professional consultant and even putting me in contact with an endocrinologist partner were invaluable in starting the Lynchburg Endocrinology and Rheumatology Clinic on July 9, 1979.

While there is some debate whether the term "stagnant" was used by my mother-in-law, the reactions of family and friends to setting up practice in Lynchburg were sobering. Between the time of our decision in late spring of 1978 and starting practice the following July, Lynchburg was in the news related to the Three Mile Island nuclear disaster involving reactors manufactured by Babcock and Wilcox, a major Lynchburg employer. Reverend Jerry Falwell was becoming a prominent national figure with his Moral Majority and there was the continued confusion of Lynchburg, Virginia, as the home of Jack Daniels Whiskey—which, of course, is Lynchburg, Tennessee. An article came out in the *Chicago Tribune* describing Lynchburg as "a town stuck in the fifties, and the people like it that way." This did not discourage Sandra or me at all. We were wary of towns growing rapidly where most realtors showing us around assumed our children would go to private schools. Sandra had grown up in Charlotte and we felt that a city's growing pains included more teenage problems with alcohol and drugs. A town stuck in the fifties? Okay!

My friends in training wondered about the appeal. Was I joining a clinic that offered a great starting salary with all moving expenses paid and help with financing a home? No, I would set up practice on my own. Were med school and college debts being paid off? No. I had worked part-time as an attendant on the psychiatry unit at Duke as an undergraduate and spent every sixth night during medical school at Duke Hospital working in the blood bank. I had no debt. With a "no" answer to all questions, they were even more puzzled. What was the allure?

Natural resources, including the setting along the James River at the foothills of our mountains, recreational activities such as hiking and fishing attracted us, as well as a viable public education system, excellent colleges and universities offering programs and adult learning possibilities and a welcoming medical community. We felt somewhat reassured in our decision when Drs. Robert and Janet Hickman, fellow Duke trainees, decided to come to Lynchburg as well.

So, how did things work out? Bob Hickman and I felt some apprehension in setting up our own practices. Janet joined the established dermatology practice of the Whitmore's—Charles and Claire. For the first three months, I simply went up the hill to Central Fidelity Bank to borrow money from our banker, Louis Stinnett, to pay my staff and office overhead. Sandra and I were down to $1200 in our bank account when I brought my first check home from the practice. I remember running into Bob Hickman at the hospital, who, likewise, was taking his first check home. We were elated.

About this time, a clinical rheumatology position opened up at Duke and my former division chief, Dr. Ralph Synderman, asked me to consider coming back. I felt that we should look at the opportunity, but Sandra, in spite of almost no money from the practice, already loved Lynchburg and did not want to go back to Duke. And she was right. Lynchburg proved to be a wonderful place to practice and raise our family.

For the first several years of practice, however, I continued to hear from a friend who set up his rheumatology practice in Atlanta. "Leave that backward little Virginia town and join me in Hotlanta." With a daughter and grandson now living in the Atlanta area, I am reminded several times each year why I love Lynchburg. As Atlanta has continued to grow, my friend makes a daily forty-five minute to one-hour commute to his office in bumper to bumper traffic. I contrast that with the seven-to-eight minute trips from home to office or hospital in the suburban setting I enjoyed for thirty-five years.

Our decision was confirmed after several years when my mother-in-law became a Lynchburg convert. The late Tom Jones contributed to that. As many Lynchburgers remember, Tom Jones owned a unique pharmacy. He was a dedicated people person and pharmacist. He listed his home phone number for emergencies and often met people at the Boonsboro store on holidays or at night, when the pharmacy was closed, to fill urgently needed prescriptions. He maintained the right focus on caring for his clientele. Often, when I returned from vacation, I found calls from Tom on the answering machine. "Dr. Jeff, Mrs. Smith ran out of refills on her methotrexate while you were gone, so I refilled that for her. I knew you wouldn't mind." Doing the right thing for the right reason.

Somehow, whatever you needed was somewhere in that store. My mother-in-law was charmed by Tom's affable nature and always seemed to find an item she could not get in Charlotte. Clothing stores and gift shops at the Boonsboro Shopping Center were also frequented during the visits. The Farm Basket was such a favorite that I bought her a sketch of the Farm Basket as a Christmas gift. Lynchburg had become a gem and "that stagnant little Virginia town" disappeared.

# "I'M NOT TAKING PREDNISONE, IT KILLED AUNT SADIE"

## (Steroids and Prednisone)

For the past four months, Carolyn had bounced around from doctor to doctor. New headaches prompted a neurology evaluation and a normal brain MRI; a migraine variant was suspected. Pain in her jaw while eating was diagnosed as TMJ (temporomandibular joint) syndrome, unrelieved by muscle relaxants and a dental guard at night. Facial pain resulted in several courses of antibiotics prescribed by her ENT doctor for possible sinusitis, but there was no improvement. She had stiffness in her shoulders and hips for several hours each morning.

After checking the patient's vital signs, our excellent office nurse, Jean Henry, came out of the exam room alarmed. "I can barely feel a pulse and can't hear a blood pressure in either arm!" It was a tip-off to the diagnosis. The patient had pulseless disease as an unusual manifestation of temporal arteritis.

Temporal arteritis (or Giant Cell Arteritis) often presents in patients over fifty years old with new headaches, scalp or facial tenderness, morning stiffness in shoulders and hips, and pain in the mouth while eating (chewing claudication). It is one of the true rheumatologic emergencies. Untreated, the patient may have sudden blindness, stroke, or death. The sedimentation rate (a measure of inflammation) is greater than 50 mm/hr. in these patients, and Carolyn waited while we ran the test. Her sed rate was 83 mm/hr. (normal 0 to 12 mm/hr.), almost certainly confirming the diagnosis.

I was eager to start treatment immediately with prednisone 20 to 30 mg twice a day. Hopefully, this would prevent a stroke or blindness. Prednisone is the specific therapy for temporal arteritis. No other medicine is an effective alternative. But Carolyn refused to take it, "I'm not taking prednisone. It killed Aunt

Sadie." Most likely Aunt Sadie had prednisone as part of a chemotherapy regimen for advanced cancer. I warned the patient of possible catastrophic consequences: stroke, blindness, or death. But she left the office determined not to take prednisone. I felt like she was a ticking time bomb. While doctors make recommendations, patients have the right to make decisions, even wrong ones.

There are some unique things about practicing medicine in Lynchburg. The size of our Central Virginia community allows us to encounter our patients everywhere. Years ago, as managed care was being debated in our country, the Lynchburg Academy of Medicine, under the guidance of presidents Dr. George Hurt and Dr. Eric Sorenson, hired Charles Hooks Associates to examine health care costs in our community. An independent study group (Tayloe Murphy) out of UVa found that without merged hospitals, HMOs (Health Maintenance Organizations), PPOs (Preferred Provider Organizations), IPAs (Independent Physician Associations), or PHOs (Physician Hospital Organizations, like Piedmont Community Health Plan), we had the next to lowest health care costs in the state. Few doctors participated with the health insurance programs and no one had their care restricted by any health care organization.

I always thought that we had a responsibility to be reasonable in our fees. The late Dr. George Craddock often addressed his patient as "friend" and once pointed out to me that while you can shear a sheep several times, you can only fleece it once. Lesson learned. I still feel that one of the greatest mistakes made by the Academy was terminating the services of Charles Hooks. He helped us deliver a message that the doctor-patient relationship is special. When I see on a TV ad that a father's opportunity to attend his daughter's wedding in face of prostate cancer begins with Centra, I cringe. Our godfather of medicine at Duke Med School, Dr. Eugene Stead, Jr., often said, "What this patient needs is a doctor." When a seriously ill patient rushes into the ER he asks for a doctor, not a hospital system or hospital administrator. Medical care begins with the patient-doctor encounter.

My admonitions regarding the risk of serious sequelae from untreated temporal arteritis did not convince Carolyn to take prednisone. Fortunately, she was close friends with the widow of one of our finest physicians. When her friend inquired about the appointment and learned about Carolyn's refusal to follow my recommendation for prednisone therapy, her response was terse and definite, "Call him back and do exactly what he says." A friend's influence rather than medical science carried the day. Over the next two years, pulses returned, blood pressure could be detected, and blindness, stroke, and death were avoided. Carolyn eventually tapered off all the prednisone.

While prednisone at times can be an effective, life-saving medicine, the majority of my female patients think prednisone does only one thing—"it makes you gain weight, doesn't it!" More an angry declaration than a question. I point out to the patient that it's a tiny, bitter-tasting pill that weighs almost nothing. There is little consolation in acknowledging the unfairness of giving her the world's best appetite stimulant and reassuring her that she won't gain weight if she doesn't overeat. True, but a harsh reality.

How did prednisone (cortisone, steroids) get such a bad rap? It was introduced into clinical medicine in 1949 by Dr. Phil Hench of the Mayo Clinic. At that time arthritis was defined as either inflammatory (rheumatoid arthritis) or non-inflammatory (osteoarthritis). If the rheumatoid arthritis (RA) patient could not tolerate gold shots (yes, real gold) or twelve to sixteen aspirins a day, there was little left to offer. Cortisone had dramatic, life-altering effects for many patients who had failed treatments available at that time. Physicians felt they had found the specific cure for RA. However, there was no experience in dosing the new medicine. If a little was good, more would probably be better. Over the next few years, side effects of steroids appeared: cataracts, bruising, softening of bones, osteoporosis, fractures, diabetes, moon face changes, weakened muscles, and even psychosis at high doses.

In academic medicine, the pendulum swings widely. Things are either all good or all bad. Today's darling is tomorrow's red-haired bastard at the family reunion. Seeing the side effects of steroids, the mantra became, "Don't give your patients steroids, they don't know how to handle them." Well, it wasn't the patients; we physicians did not know how to handle them.

Since 1949, the question has been, "What is a low dose of prednisone? What is a safe dose?" Like so many things, it's not an "all or none" scenario. Some guidance comes from a recently published review by Dr. Ted Pincus, an academic rheumatologist of the same vintage as myself. In reviewing over thirty years of practice experience, he noted a large number of RA patients chronically on 3 to 5 mg of prednisone daily for several decades, in some cases. There were few side effects. My experience was similar. In today's medical world, we are able to correct side effects like accelerated cataract development, monitor bone densities for osteoporosis and treat with appropriate meds, and use stomach protecting meds like omeprazole while avoiding concurrent NSAIDs (Non-Steroidal Anti-Inflammatory Drugs) like ibuprofen or naproxen.

So, while physicians can use steroids more safely and effectively than ever for our patients, the only thing I'll never be able to do is convince my female patients that prednisone does not make you gain weight. I expect the Nobel Prize in Medicine if I accomplish that.

# "I'VE BEEN SEEING YOU FOR SO LONG, I CAN REMEMBER WHEN YOU WERE GOOD LOOKING"

## (Doctor's Appearance)

Wow! I had been caring for Shirley more than twenty-five years. She is over eighty years old and I prefer to edit her comment to: "I remember when you were more *youthful* looking." In contrast, many patients returning to the practice after several years' absence have mentioned how I never seem to change over time. While I prefer the latter observation, I suspect things are somewhere between the two extremes.

Another long-time patient said, "I know you color your hair." Familiarity does not necessarily breed contempt. Instead, it gives the patient a right to some personal observations and license to throw a few good natured barbs at the doctor. I simply referred her to Sandra, my wife and hairstylist. Sandra has cut my hair for over forty years of our marriage. I point out that while she is of Greek extract (her family name was Lymberis), as a barber she is not Grecian (Formula)—if you get my drift. The haircutting routine began early in marriage, extending through med school, internship, residency, fellowship and practice. It was based on two ideas: efficiency and economy. Without a doubt, efficiency has been achieved. Economy has been a divided issue. While I have saved greatly on my haircuts, my naïveté was demonstrated by an estimation that the savings on my haircuts would pay for my wife and two daughters' haircuts. I believe the savings may have paid for one haircut, one time, among the three.

I have been blessed with a full head of hair from Dad's side (my maternal grandfather, Pop Hartman, was bald) and the persistence of color I attribute to Mom, whose hair did not turn gray until well into her seventies. Maybe West Virginia water running in our blood has something to do with it. A full head of hair with its original color is a great conversation piece at high school, college, and med school reunions. I've had classmates at all levels grab my hair as a toupee testing and mutter—"I don't care what they say, his hair is colored." So be it.

Youthful appearance can be disconcerting for some patients. As a senior physician, I understand the "Doogie Howser" observation—"*This person can't possibly be old enough to be a doctor!*" I remember the first time I met Dr. David Harman in the mid-1980s. He was working with Dr. Parker Lee out of a tiny office and I had arranged for my mother to come out of West Virginia for consultation regarding cataract surgery. Dave came to the waiting room to greet mother, Sandra, and me. When he left, we looked at each other with the same surprised query, "How old do you think he is?" Very young looking. For many patients, a little gray hair on their doctor is comforting. It reassures them that their physician is experienced.

During the time of medical school and specialty training through the 1970s, however, there was a trend to divest traditional images of the profession. Doctors were to dress more casually like their patients. It was felt that you might relate better on a personal basis. There was even a syndicated newspaper series by "Dr. Hip,"—how to be contemporary and cool in your patient interactions. Maybe the patients wanted a physician friend rather than an authoritative father figure. Medical students were less inclined to wear their white coats or introduce themselves as doctor or student doctor.

This was also a time of rock concerts popularized by the great Woodstock gathering. An interesting study was conducted during one of the music festivals. With the mix of youth, summer heat, alcohol, and drugs, there was always a need for medical care. Two tents were set up to care for sick attendees. One tent was staffed with traditional medical personnel—physicians and nurses in white coats and uniforms. The other tent was staffed with a medical team in contemporary clothes: jeans, tie-dyed T shirts, and sandals. If the person needed medical care he or she usually opted for the tent with the traditional medical team.

When they were sick, they wanted a doctor, not a contemporary friend.

I started practice in Lynchburg on July 9, 1979. At that time there was an unstated but understood dress code. Men wore a sport jacket, shirt and tie, with nice slacks when you made hospital rounds. At the office, the sport jacket was exchanged for a short or long white coat. The most common combination was the Navy blue blazer and khaki slacks. University of Virginia (UVa) influence showed up frequently as an orange and blue tie. Patients and fellow physicians took notice of your dress. The late Dr. William Barney relates a story in "Hello, Friend" (compiled stories about Dr. George Craddock, Warwick House Publishers, 1989, out of print). Dr. Barney had received a pair of orange slacks as a Christmas gift from his sons. He wore his new bright orange UVa pants on rounds. When he encountered Dr. Craddock at the hospital, George looked at Bill's outfit and simply said, "Bill, I like your coat." Enough said.

A dress code is certainly ancient history now in hospital and office. Things are different, but I'm not sure better. For some patients, there is still a comfort felt with the appearance of a physician in a white coat.

# "DON'T GET AN iPHONE, DR. WILSON"

I had taken care of Ms. M for over thirty years. We knew each other well. Like so many of my patients, when she heard that our practice was ending because of health problems affecting my family, she was concerned. My wife, Sandra, has breast cancer and I was diagnosed with an early onset of Parkinson's disease.

Sandra's breast cancer has an excellent prognosis. A small localized area of involvement treated with lumpectomy by Dr. Peter Plock, followed by chemotherapy and radiation therapy in the hands of Dr. Cecilia MacCallum and Dr. Joy Hilliard, leaves us optimistic for a cure.

In the fall of 2014, as my practice was winding down, Sandra and I attended our respective fifty-year high school reunions. The first Friday evening of each event involved a general gathering in a crowded venue with drinks and a band playing music too loud for our age-impaired hearing. At the Myers Park reunion in Charlotte, several classmates commented that Sandra looked the same as in high school. "That's what cancer will do for you," she responded. "It's a wig and I've lost twenty-five pounds due to chemo."

The second day of each reunion involved outdoor activities in warm weather. A wig was too hot, so Sandra wore a cap over her bald head. It's like a calling card. Instead of a sisterhood of the traveling pants, it's the sisterhood of the baseball cap. She received a similar reception at both reunions. Fellow breast cancer patients approached her with kind and warm words of encouragement and empathy. We have now witnessed this from perfect strangers when out in the Lynchburg community. My patients pray for her recovery. One patient runs a hair dresser's operation and was eager to let Sandra know that they had some wigs that were not too heavy or hot.

In August, I was diagnosed with an early onset Parkinson's disease. There is something disconcerting and bothersome about your doctor being sick. He is supposed to be giving care, not receiving it. I have been privileged to have a magnificent group of patients in my practice, some for over thirty years. We have formed personal, as well as professional, bonds. Many have included Sandra and me in their prayers. We believe in intercessory prayer and are most grateful for this. Some patients brought gifts and food. Again, most appreciated.

But Ms. M wanted to share even more. Her husband had developed a significant tremor over the years, probably related to an inherited familial condition. As his mobile phone had become dated, they purchased an I-Phone. With his tremor, however, there was a problem using the many features. As she humorously observed, at the end of the first afternoon with his I-Phone, they had no idea how many foreign phone calls they had accidentally made. They returned to their prior mobile phone.

Knowing that Parkinson's disease involves a tremor, she was being considerate, wanting me to benefit from their experience. She wanted to be part of my care. Her advice? "Don't get an I-Phone, Dr. Wilson."

Don't worry, Ms. M, I understand. I won't, and thanks for your kind and thoughtful concern.

# "I DON'T SEE HOW YOU CAN STAY IN PRACTICE"

This was a common sentiment frequently expressed by many of our patients during the last two years of the Lynchburg Rheumatology Clinic. And the answer was, I couldn't stay in practice. Closing the office over the last six months of 2010 provided time to reflect on the factors contributing to the demise of our practice.

Usually, the individual making the observation was a Medicare patient who reviewed his monthly summary statement and realized how little Medicare paid of our reasonable charges. My office business manager, Sharon Sirocco, compiled a list of our most frequent procedures and tests, comparing our charges and the amount allowed by Medicare. We were paid 66 percent of the office visit fee, 26 percent of the lab charge for sedimentation rate (of interest, a patient recently showed a bill from her evaluation at a medical center; their charge for a sed rate was ten times greater than ours) and 35 percent for a CBC (complete blood count). Bone density was reimbursed at 34 percent and a shoulder x-ray at 36 percent of charges. A sample representing office visit, lab, and x-ray charges found Medicare reimbursing us overall at 45 percent of our charges.

Meanwhile, overhead expenses were increasing. With new ownership of our office building, the realtor-owner-building manager increased our rent by 65 percent for 2010. Although we asked for a proposal of the increase in July, he delayed the proposal until mid-November leaving no time to make alternative plans. The new landlord explained that his utilities costs were going up (weren't everyone's?) and he planned to recoup those costs in the new lease. The exorbitant increase in rent for 2010 made a case for a realtor to avoid in the future in any capacity.

New regulations required software modifications for our Amicore Penchart electronic medical record (EMR). The system would have to be modified for new prescriptions submitted electronically, and we already had IT problems in operation like all EMRs, partly related to computer virus woes. It seemed that all computer-software solutions were $30,000. Reminding one of the IT techs that this was a solo operation, going out of business, elicited the reply, "Well, we've got to make a living, too." Their support and understanding have served as a benchmark for excessive IT charges common to many vendors.

For the final five years (2005 to 2010), office income decreased 5 percent each year. Our office staff (See…"You Have the Best Office") did not have a raise during that time. Considering the importance of the health matters they dealt with daily, it was ridiculous that they were earning about one-sixth of what a union auto worker was paid. Our aging patient population presented the unsustainable scenario of a greater proportion of Medicare recipients in this setting of increasing costs and decreasing compensation. We were a small practice going out of business. An editorial in the *New England Journal of Medicine* (February 12, 2009, Isaacs et al., "The Independent Physician— Going, Going") outlines the difficulties of operating a solo practice of any sort.

During that time, we informed our patients of the dilemma and solicited any recommendations in a January 2010 newsletter simply titled *HELP*. Many Medicare patients offered to pay the difference. As a Medicare participating physician you are not allowed to balance bill the patient. Some patients suggested we *stop participating with Medicare*. If I were starting a new practice, I would consider this. While that might have made good business sense, we felt it would leave our patients in a confusing administrative mess, and from an ethical standpoint it would mean ending the care of patients we had seen for over the last thirty years when they became Medicare eligible. We had previously stopped seeing Medicaid patients after twenty-five years of participation in the program when compensation was less than overhead expenses. It's one thing to do charity work for free; it's another to pay money to do it. Was the government turning the Medicare patient into a Medicaid patient? Any of my Medicare patients who had run their own business recognized our problems and began to understand the ramifications for the Medicare patient's access to care in the future.

*See more patients.* We had a full practice. In addition to scheduled visits every fifteen minutes, we had patients coming in for "lab only" visits—having blood tests to monitor strong medications like methotrexate. They often had to see the doctor as a work-in if problems had arisen. We always tried to see any unscheduled patients with urgent problems as well. The office was efficient and busy.

One patient was mystified. With demographics showing an aging population, more and more people had arthritis with ever-increasing need for rheumatology care. I explained that regardless of this correct observation, if reasonable compensation for care was not present, that need would not be met. My fellow physician, plastic surgeon Tim Silvester, illustrates the problem relating the story of two brothers running a sandwich shop. Brother Bob explained to brother Tom that it cost $5.00 to make a sandwich which they sold for $4.00. Brother Tom's answer—"We'll have to make it up with volume." With the government fixing the prices, you couldn't "make it up" by seeing more patients.

One government regulation was especially onerous for a solo practice like mine. The physician had to be on site or you could not charge for Medicare patient services. If a patient was due for a scheduled injection such as weekly methotrexate or lab only studies, these would have to be delayed if I was out of the office. Any time the office was closed, while rent and other overhead expenses continued, there was no income. This made little sense in a day of telecommunications when I could immediately be aware of complications or lab abnormalities and make appropriate adjustments within a matter of hours. Now there's interest in teleconferences where a patient is evaluated remotely with diagnosis and treatment regimens prescribed. Even intensive care patients, with life threatening illnesses, may be monitored remotely. Required on-site patient service is an archaic regulation, which certainly hindered the viability of our practice. Now there are television ads for pharmacy chains establishing urgent care nurse practitioner clinics and providing flu and shingles vaccinations. I wonder how they get around on-site regulations. I suspect it is by a non-participating status or more political clout than a solo practitioner.

*Work longer hours and take less time off.* Don't mention this to my wife. In thirty-five years of practice, we had a handful of two-week vacations and perhaps one vacation that was longer than two weeks. It is her pet peeve which produces a recurring siren's song—"Just quit and retire, so we can travel." Indeed, a published study showed that doctors initially *did* work longer hours ("Trends in the Work Hours of Physicians in the United States," *Journal of the American Medical Association; Vol* 303; 747; February 24, 2010). It resulted in less time for educational programs (both local and national medical meetings) as well as less participation in health departments, free clinics, and medical missionary work. Something's got to give.

*You have too many employees.* This observation allowed me to remember the halcyon days of early practice in the 1980s. Our office, like many, had a front office receptionist/business manager and a back office clinical person to check in patients and assist with clinical procedures and treatments. Accounting was with the Pegboard system. The patient had a bill for that visit as they left the office as well as return appointment information. It was estimated that an office needed two staff members/doctor. As our office grew from a two-man office, employees were added to provide more services such as in-office lab and x-ray. These were revenue generating additions.

Now it is estimated that an office needs six support staff per physician. What changed? Regulation. Starting practice in 1979, our business advisor presented us with a twenty-eight page folder of federal and state guidelines for running a medical business. Regulations in the medical field have expanded like the Federal Registry. Over the years, compliance with OSHA, CLIA, COLA, HIPAA, and now EMR guidelines have slowed productivity and increased overhead without generating additional income. When closing my office, I had over 1,000 pages of manuals related to these entities—manuals I have to store for seven years if clinically related and five years for business related records.

*Recruit another rheumatologist.* The average age of a rheumatologist in our country is fifty-four years. The young physicians are tuned in to the remunerative differences in more highly procedural specialties. Several years ago, a local Lynchburg man just finishing medical school spent a two-week clinical rotation at our rheumatology practice. He was inclined toward rheumatology, and I fantasized having him join the practice about the time I might slow down or retire. Although he had a good experience on a rheumatology rotation as an intern, he called one night and asked, in effect, if we had a procedure in rheumatology where we zapped someone with a laser at $1,000 a treatment. Not exactly, I admitted. He is now a successful ophthalmologist.

A rheumatology friend in Roanoke Rapids, North Carolina, repeated a familiar scenario experienced by many solo or small practice rheumatologists. The young rheumatologist recruited at a guaranteed salary for a specified year or two would be reluctant to buy into the practice when he realized he might be making less money in the face of decreasing compensation. Going to another practice meant leaving the original rheumatologist with the burden of additional patients for an already full practice. I don't fault the young rheumatologists with their decisions, and I would not recommend coming into a small practice like mine. Large clinics or hospital systems could offer greater recruiting incentives such as help paying off training debts (up to $250,000 in many cases) and providing economies of scale.

*Join a larger group.* I investigated this possibility with two groups. One group analyzed our practice and felt that if I joined them it would significantly increase my income, but there was not room for my staff. We decided to sink or swim together. The other group recruited a newly trained young rheumatologist and, although they had interest in my staff, they did not have a place for me. I would not have blamed my staff for looking at work opportunities with this larger clinic, but they had the same feeling. All or none. So Lynchburg Rheumatology Clinic which opened its practice July 9, 1979, closed its doors December 31, 2010.

Saying goodbye to patients was no fun. The administrative requirements of scanning records and providing x-rays and summary notes plus disposing of office furnishings and x-ray equipment was a hassle and we had to stop seeing patients for the last month of practice. Closing a practice in 2010 was much harder than opening a practice in 1979. But the worst part was seeing the patients for the last time. These were tearful goodbyes shared by office staff, patients, and their doctor. As our staff left that last day, I never would have expected that starting in July, our rheumatology practice would be reborn.

# "YOU SHOULDN'T HAVE ORDERED THAT TEST"
## (Polymyalgia Rheumatica)

My seventy-nine-year-old patient was fussing at me during his follow-up visit. Two weeks earlier he presented for evaluation of diffuse aches and pains in joints and muscles. I hoped he had polymyalgia rheumatic (PMR), an inflammatory illness that occurs in patients over fifty years of age with sedimentation rates greater than 50 mm/hr and marked morning stiffness in shoulders and hips. This often comes on suddenly and the patient feels like he (or she) aged twenty years overnight.

Why would I hope for this diagnosis? Because it is exquisitely sensitive to low dose prednisone and usually has a limited duration over eighteen months to two years. The return visit is especially gratifying as the patient's symptoms are markedly improved, often after the first prednisone tablet. Indeed, my patient was greatly improved, but griping about the PSA test.

I always emphasize to my patients at the initial visit that PMR is a diagnosis of exclusion. Since it occurs in our older population, there is always concern that an underlying tumor or cancer may be presenting with these aches and pains. In all patients, I check a serum protein electrophoresis to rule out underlying myeloma bone cancer and, in the male patient, I check the PSA (prostate specific antigen). Apparently, Medicare did not think a rheumatologist should be checking the PSA and did not want to pay for the test. The patient agreed, "You shouldn't have ordered that test." If Medicare didn't want to pay for the test, it should not be done.

The patient's PSA level was 134.2 ng/ml (normal <4.0). His symptoms were caused by metastatic prostate cancer. I stopped his prednisone and directed him toward urology and oncology evaluations. If the PSA had not been checked, the diagnosis and appropriate treatment would have been missed or delayed.

But what a worrisome mindset. If Medicare or the patient's health plan doesn't want to pay for a test, one might think it's not *important*. Our patients need to examine motivation for denial of a claim. As a physician, I was paid nothing when ordering sophisticated blood tests such as a PSA or protein electrophoresis or specialized radiology studies such as CT scans or MRIs. These tests were ordered to provide a thorough evaluation and the best care. What is the interest of Medicare or the health plan? I would contend that these organizations are interested more in the bottom line. Delaying or restricting care may decrease health care costs, but rarely benefit patients.

However, once patients believe that Medicare or their health plan knows what's best for diagnosis and treatment, they're certainly ready for socialized medicine…and a different physician.

# "YOUR FATHER TOOK CARE OF MY MOTHER"
## (Immunogenetics, HLA B27, Autoimmunity, ANA Test, Agent Orange, Vitamin D)

My seventy-eight-year-old patient remembered that twenty years earlier his mother was treated at the Lynchburg Rheumatology Clinic for temporal arteritis, the same condition he had now developed. But my father was not a doctor. I had taken care of his mother when I was in my late thirties and the patient was in his late fifties at the time. Either I looked pretty old then or I had aged well. Preferring to believe the latter, I explained that PMR (Polymyalgia rheumatica) and temporal arteritis (giant cell arteritis) tend to run in families, like so many of our rheumatologic conditions.

Probably the best example of inheritance and a model for many diseases is the HLA B27 story. In the late 1960s, before extensive histocompatibility (HLA) testing was being performed for transplantation research, a report in one of our medical journals (Noer, HR: An "experimental" epidemic of Reiter's syndrome JAMA [*Journal of the American Medical Association*] 198: 693-698, 1966) described an outbreak of Shigella dysentery on a Navy cruiser. It was not unusual that a large number of the crew (602 out of 1276) would be affected by this infectious diarrhea and most would recover in a few days. However, ten of the sailors developed an on-going chronic inflammatory condition (Reiter's Syndrome) with features of arthritis, conjunctivitis (eye inflammation) and urethritis (inflammation in the urinary tract). The infectious process had triggered a persistent inflammatory illness.

In the 1970s, histocompatibility was being investigated. If two individuals had a similar makeup—for instance HLA A1; B27; C3; D4—then they would be a match—and most likely transplantation of organs from one to the other would be compatible and not rejected. As data were compiled, we found that the incidence of HLA B27 was 4 to 8 percent in the general population, but 96 percent in patients with the prototypical spondyloarthropathy condition ankylosing spondylitis, and 50 to 60 percent in patients with Reiter's Syndrome. Other diseases seen more frequently in families positive for HLA B27 include psoriasis, iritis/uveitis (inflammatory eye diseases) and inflammatory bowel diseases such as Crohn's disease. The individual patient might have one of these disorders or a combination.

In a classic follow-up article (Calin, A; Fries, JF: An "Experimental" Epidemic of Reiter's Syndrome Revisited; *Annals of Internal Medicine* 84: 564-566, 1976), five of the original ten patients were located. All but one were B27 positive, a strong correlation. The four B27 positive sailors had persistent, active Reiter's, while the one who was B27 negative had minimal disease activity.

HLA B27 is part of the individual's inherited immunogenetic makeup. It never changes. A blood test shows if the patient is HLA B27 positive or negative. An important study in the late 1970s clarified the significance of B27 positivity. Blood donors with no active health problems were tested. Individuals positive for B27 were followed over the next two decades. Only 20 percent developed a B27 associated disease. Having an inherited immunogenetic makeup that includes HLA B27 does not doom the patient for the development of a particular disease. It simply provides the setting for these disorders to be triggered. In the case of the Navy sailors and many patients, an infection acted as the trigger.

Prior to this, rheumatic fever was the best known example of an autoimmune disease triggered by an infection. In some patients after the eradication of a strep infection, the immune system seemed misdirected. As part of its surveillance function, the immune system would begin to react against the patient's joints, skin, and heart—an autoimmune reaction resulting in rheumatic fever. The infection was gone, but once the immune system was turned on, it began to react against self (autoimmune).

Infectious processes have been the primary suspects as triggers for these diseases. However, a study reported in the *New England Journal of Medicine* (Ayele, FT et al., HLA Class II Locus and Susceptibility to Podoconiosis; *NEJM*, 366; 13 March 29, 2012) raises other possibilities. Members of a tribe in Ethiopia, with similar immunogenetics demonstrated by human genome mapping, developed a disease mimicking elephantiasis. The classic elephantiasis (remember pictures in the *National Geographic* magazine of the natives with massively swollen lower legs?) is an infectious disease caused by a parasite Wucheria bancrofti. But in the case of these Ethiopian patients, the disease is triggered by walking on volcanic red clay. Mineral particles absorbed through their feet trigger off podoconiosis— a disease looking just like elephantiasis. The lesson? Environmental factors may play a role as triggers for varied diseases in the immunogenetically predisposed individual, and our environment may be getting less friendly.

I became more suspicious of environmental triggers during the 1980s. I began to follow three patients with atypical clinical features of lupus—all were white, two of the three were male, and all died. Usually, we thought of lupus as a disease of young black females. Although the old Merck Manual of the late 1960s defined lupus as an "invariably fatal disease related to tuberculosis," this was completely wrong and we did not expect a high mortality rate, especially after a short duration of the disease and modern treatment with steroids and medicines like hydroxychloroquine (Plaquenil). The family history of two patients suggested an inherited tendency toward autoimmune diseases like lupus. The sister of my one female patient had rheumatoid arthritis and was followed at my practice. The female cousin of one male patient (TJ) had polymyositis—an inflammatory muscle disorder now in remission. She was also followed in my practice.

The three patients were Vietnam War veterans, and the common feature in each case was exposure to Agent Orange. Since that time, an increased incidence of lymphoma has been related to Agent Orange, and TJ, who had an unusual complication of aseptic necrosis requiring bilateral hip replacements, died at the VA Hospital with a rare small intestinal lymphoma. His daughter was subsequently diagnosed with lupus. The one female patient was a nurse on the front line in Vietnam with Agent Orange exposure mainly from wounded patients. Autoimmune sequelae of Agent Orange are being increasingly recognized in these veterans and in their progeny. The effect of Agent Orange is probably an example of epigenetics in which the chemical agent causes a change in the DNA which is passed on. This is discussed in a book by Lynda Van Devanter (deceased) *Home Before Morning: The Story of an Army Nurse in Vietnam* (2001). The other male patient had active renal disease from his lupus and died with an unusual complication of pulmonary hemorrhaging.

Our Vietnam Veterans are dying off, but a caveat remains. When patients associate the onset of an illness to things like moving into a new house ("sick house") or exposures in the work environment or following a procedure like silicone breast implants, we need to pay attention. We are probably seeing a person with predisposed immunogenetics having a disease triggered by an environmental factor. For years, I resisted this idea, especially with regard to silicone breast implants causing autoimmune disease. An excellent book, *Science on Trial* by Marcia Angell, MD, chronicles the evolution of the suspected association to greed stimulated legal actions. While the academic medical centers found no evidence of an association of silicone breast implants causing connective tissue disease, I remain suspicious that environmental triggers in the immunogenetically predisposed individual may still cause diseases like lupus.

With a host of potential infectious or environmental triggers in the setting of inherited immunogenetics, the question is whether anything can prevent the development of these diseases. Each week I would see several patients referred for rheumatology evaluation because they had a positive ANA (Antinuclear Antibody) test. The patients were often alarmed when told by their physician, or informed via the internet, that this is associated with lupus or scleroderma or other related connective tissue diseases such as polymyositis and Sjögren's Syndrome. But this is a very sensitive test (that is, a lot of false positive tests) and we know that the diagnosis of lupus or any connective tissue disease depends on a set of diagnostic criteria being met—the ANA test being representative of only one criterion and never diagnostic by itself.

For the last ten years, I have been interested in the potential for vitamin D and Plaquenil (hydroxychloroquine) to have an immunomodulatory effect in these patients. Most of these patients have extremely low vitamin D levels. While we don't want to suppress the immune system so much that it doesn't handle infections, we would like to stop its over-reaction causing autoimmune diseases like lupus—that is, modulate the immune system. Many of these ANA (+) patients who did not fulfill diagnostic criteria for definite lupus or related connective tissue disease were followed for two to three years with vitamin D replacement to levels of 50 to 60 ng/ml and hydroxychloroquine. Not only did they fail to develop active lupus or associated disease, but the ANA tests became negative. Although the sensitive ANA tests may have many false positives, when it's negative, it really helps to rule out these diseases.

At this time, the prospects for altering the inherited immunogenetics or eliminating infectious and environmental triggers seem unlikely. But could we decrease the likelihood of the individual patient developing these diseases by altering factors such as vitamin D deficiency? In the June 2007 *Arthritis & Rheumatism* journal article entitled "Are We at a Stage to Predict Autoimmune Rheumatic Diseases?" the author writes: "The capability of prediction will be valuable only if preventive measures can be adopted. Knowledge is accumulating to recommend avoidance of exposure to UV light, specific diet, avoidance of specific chemicals (silica, Mercury, toxic oil, and the like [I would add Agent Orange]), use of specific contraceptives or vaccines, and based on animal studies, administration of vitamin D." A more recent interesting article was reported in the April 10, 2012, *Rheumatology News* suggesting that the detection and treatment of vitamin D deficiency may help prevent development of autoimmune diseases. The investigator, Dr. Carol A. Hitchon, presented her findings at the annual meeting of the Canadian Rheumatology Association. Accumulating data suggest that vitamin D plays a role in maintaining both tolerance and immunity to pathogens. "If you are deficient in vitamin D, it may lead to a break of self-tolerance and the development of autoimmunity. Similarly, deficient vitamin D can impair or alter the initial response to pathogens, leading to increased microbial load, which can also increase or affect autoimmunity." I ask my patients, who are vitamin D deficient, to be the champion in their family, going after members of the next generation to detect and correct vitamin D deficiency. Perhaps we can prevent some of these diseases.

What does the future hold? I predict that eventually at birth the individual's genomic mapping will identify the inherited disease tendencies. Infectious disease triggers for the individual's particular genetic makeup will call for a set of specific vaccines to be provided, and environmental triggers to be avoided will be identified. Improved health care and honest health care savings will be achieved, not by restricting care and payments, but by true prevention of disease.

# "YOU HAVE THE BEST OFFICE"

What they meant was "...you have the best office *staff*." We were all complimented and I was personally gratified when patients frequently shared this observation with us, and they were right. It was a special group of people who made my last years of practice at the Lynchburg Rheumatology Clinic (LRC—pronounced "lerk") a great success. By "success" I mean a definition offered on an interview with Bill Gates and Warren Buffett. They defined success as being able to do the work you want to do with people who care about each other. Scarlet Dewitt, Dee Gresham, Sharon Sirocco, Jeanette Witt, Jean Henry, and Lori McDaniel provided this setting for me.

It probably surprised the drug company representative sponsoring a lunchtime meeting at the clinic when I mentioned that there was love in our office. As I explained, C. S. Lewis wrote about *The Four Loves* and we daily witnessed affection, friendship, and charity in our concerns about each other and our patients. So, there's the scandal in our office, not exactly reality show material, but the basis of unique relationships resulting in "the best office." *Our Health* magazine each year recognizes "Best Bedside Manner" in varied medical specialties. LRC received this award, and like Christmas gifts and goodies kindly and thoughtfully provided by our patients, it is a recognition of that remarkable group of friends making up our office staff.

Let me tell you about LRC's Angels. **Scarlet**—the employee who was with me the longest, started October 1980 as a nineteen-year-old blonde (natural, I thought). I had the pleasure of watching her mature into an amazing wife, mother, daughter, and even grandmother. Scarlet was the point guard at LRC. Her first impression about patients from the initial phone contact or patient encounter was uncanny. The knowledge and concern she had for our entire patient population was remarkable. And, yet, she's the employee who almost died at the office. How

45

could that be? Because I almost killed her April 1st several years ago. I was on call for hospital consults when Scarlet notified me that a consult had been called in on a prior patient who had been dismissed from the practice—a disagreeable fellow whom I hoped never to deal with again. I fumed all day—"Contact the referring doctor. Tell him someone else will have to see that jerk. Are you sure it's not someone else with the same name?" No, no, I was assured it was the individual I dreaded. Not till the end of the day as the office was closing did my point guard say: "Incidentally, you don't have a consult—April fool!" It would have been justifiable homicide!

However, being a mature, responsible person, I chose to get even rather than murder. A year or so later, the morning after a dental appointment for a molar extraction following a root canal, I came into the office and went to the front desk. I slurred an explanation, barely moving my mouth. "Tell the patients I can't talk much today—the dentist broke my jaw when he removed the tooth," I mumbled. Well, Scarlet immediately got up and headed through the kitchen and across the hall. She was crying, so upset by what had happened. When she returned, I said with clear enunciation, "Actually, I feel much better. I think I'll be fine. April fool!" I'm still a *little* sorry I did that, but it showed the dedication and concern of this magnificent person.

Over the years, this concern was demonstrated again and again. I will always remember the incident when an irate husband accosted Scarlet at the front office window to the waiting room. He was angry that his wife had developed a heart condition and blamed us. For years, we always responded to any worsening of her health, working her into the office schedule multiple times and hospitalizing her with varied complaints, sometimes diagnosing ailments with subtle presenting symptoms. Scarlet knew this and, after he left, she was in tears, struck by the anger of the husband and lack of appreciation for the special care and consideration his wife had received. The incident told me a lot about the patient and her husband, but, most importantly, even more about Scarlet.

If you want to get an idea of the value of an individual to the office, listen to what others say. At one point, Scarlet was having an altercation with the acting managing physician. As office relations between the two came to a boil, Lori, who had only been with us a short time, said, "Whatever you do, don't let Scarlet quit."

Scarlet and I share the same wedding anniversary date—June 20th. Blake Dewitt has been like an extra bonus with Scarlet. When we needed help evaluating an office or home remodeling project, we could always count on reliable, sound advice and help from Blake. Watching Blake develop his construction company over the years has been almost as rewarding as watching Scarlet develop into such a magnificent person.

**Dee**—The most intelligent, multi-talented person who ever worked at LRC (doctors included) is Dee Gresham, starting with LRC in 1982. She was unparalleled as a lab tech. After CVTC training, she could get blood out of a stone or draw blood from a moving target. Patients would ask if Dee was working the day they needed blood drawn, especially if they were difficult sticks. More importantly, when Dee thought something was suspicious about a patient or their lab, you paid attention. Years ago, we had a young lady with suspicious cells in her peripheral blood film. I wasted time and money sending the slide for review by pathology. "Reactive lymphocytes" was their interpretation. No help. I hospitalized the patient and discovered she had an unusual breast lymphoma and these were circulating lymphoma cells in her peripheral blood. Dee just knew something wasn't right about them.

When COLA and CLIA began the government intrusion in the lab and OSHA followed in the general office, we had to establish manuals and procedures, handle controls, and still take care of patients. The first site visit and examination was stressful for all of us but, like all challenges to the office, Dee did it exceptionally well and we celebrated at my house with an "UnCOLA" party. In spite of handling the extraneous government "PITA" (pain in the assets), Dee's care for our patients remained the top priority.

Excellence in the area of their job description is just the tip of the iceberg for my office staff. For years, the office was graced with a different orchid almost weekly. Dee and her husband, Jim, compete, and win, at orchid competitions. They produce over a hundred varieties in their own greenhouse. I bet no other office had patients stop after their blood drawing and ask questions about an orchid sitting on a table in the office. Former patients still inquire about "the Orchid Lady." I may not remember the names of specific orchids but I'll never forget the story about the eighty-year-old streaker at the orchid show who received a blue ribbon for dried arrangements.

"Oh, is that a picture from Japan?" No, that's Hawaii where Dee lived when her father, Orion Templeton, was in the Navy. When you walked through the halls of LRC you saw photographs in homemade wooden frames, gratis Jim Gresham. The warmth of wood and our office color schemes were comfortable from the pictures on the walls to the large front chart rack and exam room chart holders—all enhancements by the Greshams. When special needs arose, they were always there. Jim and I spent many after-office hours hanging lead-lined sheetrock for an x-ray room, and Jim's woodworking talent is displayed in our finished basement at home.

For years Dee spearheaded our Thanksgiving hot dog fest and seasonal Christmas decorations in the office. This talented person can sketch—witness my picture from the Ten Miler race—although I contend my nose is out of proportion! Visiting her home, you'll see sketches of her son, Scott, as a youth. At Christmastime, if she drew your name for her Pollyanna, look out! Each year I asked for "World Peace" and one year my gift was a Tupperware container full of green pea soup—"World Peas." As my high school graduation Zodiac watch aged, she arranged for me to get—almost a Rolex watch—a Rolodex modified watch, which will be with me as long as the staff's over-generous Seiko gift watch. Each year she honors my mother by making "June's" peanut butter fudge. Daughter, Melissa, especially appreciates this.

When Dee mentioned going part-time, I told her she could do anything she wanted. She earned it. There was not a day you spent in the office that Dee was not there in one way or another. Her courage going through worrisome times with eye ailments was incredible. Her cares and concerns as wife and mother are part of a complete person. Her role as daughter provided us with guidance in treating our aging parents with compassion and humor. It was a treat to interact with her father and I am left with one of my favorite Thanksgiving stories. Frustrated with the kids asking for one dish after another to be passed to them, her dad finally said, "Just eat what's near you." I will always be grateful for the important part Dee played in our LRC journey.

**Sharon**—aka The Rock. Who would expect such toughness in a little package affectionately known as Munchkin, Sweet Pea, and Little Chicken? And "The Rock" doesn't just refer to improved bone density or the highest vitamin D level in the office, which she would always let us know about. It is more about the journey as she became an essential part of LRC. Sharon was hired as a transcriptionist in 1985. That position doesn't even exist in today's EMR (Electronic Medical Record) world; we have "scribes." She always wanted to learn more and assume more responsibility and gradually became our business manager. One time she listed all the things she did on a daily basis—30 items. Over the years, she became a Notary Public, certified coder, in-house IT expert, human resource manager, bookkeeper, and completed an on-line course for medical office management. She had the toughest job—bringing me the bad news as rent or overhead went up while Medicare compensation decreased. So maybe she was "The Rock" because of handling all of this.

No, not just that alone. I remember the night in October 1994 when she called, preparing to go to MCV for her kidney and pancreas transplant. She was understandably apprehensive, but you could sense her strong faith and courage as she left for Richmond starting this great adventure. After the transplant, she experienced problems with osteoporotic stress fractures, which were just beginning to be understood as a complication with transplants. Her spirit and desire to be back with us at work as soon as possible over this period of time was exemplary of a dedicated employee and an indispensable member of our LRC family. Munchkin has been more like the rock Simon Peter in faith—a strong base on which LRC rested. She would often share inspirational E-mails helpful in stressful times.

We all know of her strong spiritual faith that patients and friends witness. Sharon is more of a true mother to her nephews than most biological mothers could be. She is in touch with special needs and concerns of staff and patients of LRC. She has been my trusted adviser in many of these areas. She is a dedicated daughter and talented singer as witnessed in one memorable church Christmas program video. The hills were alive with music that day.

With each new challenge to the practice, she would rise up: prepare compliance forms for the latest extraneous government regulation (remember Red Flag Rules?), look for other possible practice venues, find less expensive liability insurance. As VPMSO (Virginia Physicians Management Service Organization) worked her toward part-time, she worried about the cost to our practice of taking her back full-time. Should she quit and look elsewhere? As I told Munchkin then, and repeat now, it was never a matter of taking her back. She was always with us then, and always will be in the future. Thanks to Sharon, Munchkin, and especially the Rock.

**Jeanette**—Sometimes the value of a clinic worker is shown in unusual ways. For instance, there was one employee whose time off was announced to me verbally or by E-mail every time she would be gone for vacation, doctor's appointment, or even just her afternoon off! Scarlet, our x-ray tech in Jeanette's absence, wanted me forewarned. Above all, don't order any foot x-rays! Jeanette (starting with LRC in 2002) is the best x-ray tech anyone could have. She sometimes enlisted help from husband, David, to keep the old x-ray unit working— holding it together with rubber bands, chicken wire, and Band-Aids, I think. But that's not why she's the best. It's her attitude and spirit. Patients and co-workers experienced the most pleasant personality to work with. Jeanette always treated the patients with the courtesy and caring our clinic intended to provide.

She is a dedicated wife, mother, and grandmother. She is a person of great faith which, I believe, enhanced her relationship with our patients. She is thoughtful and thanked me several times for getting an updated bone density machine that changed a 45-minute ordeal lying on a hard table to a quick 10 to 15-minute test. She was more thankful about the greater comfort the shortened test time provided our patients than the time it saved her. Like so many of LRC's angels, she wore more than one hat. Jeanette would check patients into the exam rooms, interview the patients, and check vital signs. When not performing her core duties as x-ray and bone density tech, she would help out in the front office. I always enjoyed overhearing her conversations with co-workers and patients about church activities and religious studies. My minister at First Presbyterian Church, John Scholer, observed in a sermon that sometimes the only religion or experience of faith some people have is what they witness in others. Jeanette walks the walk, and the patients know it. She was an important part in the development of LRC's health ministry. And you know what else? Jeanette loved my homemade Christmas granola.

**Jean**—Without a doubt, when I was back in my office or between exam rooms, the name I heard called most often was Jean. "Jean, telephone." "Jean, here's a form for you to fill out." And I did it, too. "Jean, let's do a shoulder in room one." "Band-Aid in two and show her the shoulder exercises." "Give the handouts or information on…" I would start out the day presenting Jean with a list of patients to call, based on lab reports that came in the night before, for modification of meds and most often vitamin D adjustments. She somehow would be able to call the patients during the day and explain the changes. She was educating the patients at each encounter—whether checking them into the exam room—BP, methotrexate dose, prednisone regimen, AM gel, which joints were most bothersome, updated family history, recent surgeries, etc. Her patience was tested daily with the frustrations of trying to get meds approved or prescriptions re-approved in spite of the unnecessary hurdles put up by the health insurers. It might be sufficient to say, which is true, that Jean is the best nurse I have ever worked with. Not just at LRC but in my experiences at Duke, in the Navy, or in any hospital setting.

Maybe she's the best nurse because she's one of the best people you can know: country girl, mother, grandmother, church member, dog lover, and valued friend (we loved hearing about her forays to New York visiting well-to-do friends). Jean is a person of great and tested faith. She provided dedicated terminal nursing care to her father and an elderly relative. Some people say that a gift without the giver is incomplete. The gift of being the best nurse was given at home as well as in the office.

Jean also walks the walk. A unique enhancement of our office has been the health ministry and spirituality endeavor. This would have been impossible without Jean. It began with the new patient interview when Jean would inquire about religious affiliation and provide a copy of our handout on spirituality and faith. It continued with each patient encounter afterward. Patients sensed her sincere interest in them above and beyond providing medical services. She let us know about special concerns or stresses affecting the patient. When I would pick up the chart before entering the exam room, there often was a note: "spouse sick" or "family member deceased." Frequently, patients asked us to pray for them or a relative. And, during the last year, many of the patients prayed for us as we tried to determine the future of LRC.

Jean was special, not only because she was the only red head in the office, but because she made the world's best zucchini relish.

**Lori**—Everyone should have a Hokie on his staff. When I think of Lori, I recall my patient Eugene Morris's story about taking Winnie (both Hokies) home to meet the family. His father would meet Eugene's dates over the years, and at the conclusion of the date he would usually say, "Eugene, you can do better than that." Until he brought Winnie home—"Eugene, you can't do any better than that." That applies to Lori. What a magnificent addition to our staff. The only regret is that I wish she had joined us sooner than 2003. Somehow she was able to balance the frustration dealing with Medicare and all our payers (an ever-increasing aggravation) yet maintain and project a caring and pleasant demeanor with the patient on the phone or at the check-in window of the waiting room.

She had a comprehensive, real feel for the practice from day one. Witness her observation about Scarlet during her altercation with the managing physician. I once told her that she is our "Iron Man"—like Lou Gehrig. When needs arose for others to be absent, even on an emergency basis, she was always there. Sometimes if I made a sudden change in office hours— "Let's work this Wednesday afternoon"—Lori would juggle appointments, often including her own schedule, to make things work. For instance, she would come back a day early from visiting her elderly mother in Richmond to make the office work.

Lori was quick to develop a feeling of pride and protection for our practice. She appreciated the uniqueness of our clinic and worried about the imminent demise of LRC with decreasing Medicare payments in the face of increasing regulations that always resulted in higher overhead expenses. Because of that, we were especially incensed by patients who manipulated the system or tried to stiff us. Lori was as adept as Scarlet at identifying these individuals. I remember the case of the lawyer who objected to paying for his wife's x-rays, stating that when she was seen at UVa orthopedics, the physician said our x-rays were no good and threw them in the trash. This is not an uncommon gambit to avoid paying the bill. Early in my practice, I might have been intimidated, inclined to write off that charge or forget about it. But with Lori's encouragement (insistence?), I called the chairman of orthopedics at UVa and with his help sorted out this story with the attending orthopedist. The story was not true and after I received the "trashed" x-rays back, we contacted the lawyer and let him know that either he got the story wrong—or we knew he was gaming the system (our politicians would say he misspoke; the rest of us would say he lied). We sent notes in preparation of turning his account over to the creditor service and the bill was paid. Well done, Lori!

Beyond dedication and excellence in her "job description," Lori is fun. While all the staff was up to date on current events (especially our national political scene) and TV shows like "Modern Family," "The Middle," "NCIS," "Dancing with the Stars," and "Big Bang Theory," Lori was the only staff member I could talk with about sports. This was especially fun at March Madness time. Office beach time, lake time, or afternoon lunch and a movie—she's an enthusiastic organizer and participant.

It was a special treat to vicariously enjoy her excitement and pride as son, Brad, attended and graduated from the Naval Academy and get a few glimmerings of being raised as a "Navy brat" herself. Go Navy! We shared concern after the tragic shootings at Virginia Tech and shared the joy of Ashley's wedding. Having watched my wife, Sandra, go through the scheduling and preparation details for our daughters' weddings, I could appreciate the investment of time and love she put into this big day. All Tom McDaniel and I have to do in our position is "show them the money" and watch the movie *Father of the Bride* with our daughters.

I only had to critically reprimand Lori once. Coming up to the front office I found Lori and Scarlet laughing—not an unusual occurrence. Lori had answered the phone—and instead of saying, "Dr. Wilson's office," she greeted the caller saying, "Dr. Wilson's awful." As the Managing Physician, I felt compelled to explain that this greeting would probably not encourage patients to make an appointment. Thank you, Lori, for being part of the best years of my practice.

Addendum: Since LRC closed December 31, 2010, our group continues to get together for an occasional lunch and birthday celebration. We have shared our good times and some bad times with continued concerns and love for each other. I consider LRC's Angels as extended family. I resumed practice with Rheumatology of CVFP (Central Virginia Family Physicians) July 2011, and to my good fortune and to the benefit of past and new patients, Lori McDaniel joined me as my front office manager. Our former patients still ask about each of my angels.

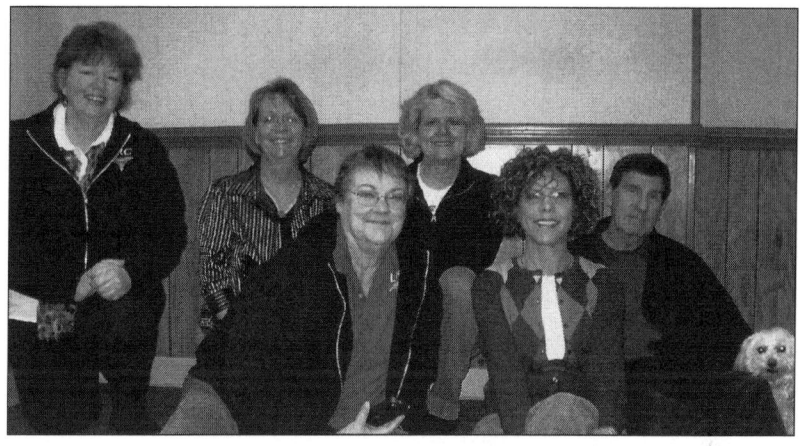

**LRC's Angels, December 31, 2010**
*Back row (left to right): Jean Henry, Jeanette Witt, Lori McDaniel,*
*Dr. Wilson and Murphy*
*Front row (left to right): Dee Gresham, Scarlet Dewitt*
*Missing: Sharon Sirocco*

# "WHAT DO YOU KNOW ABOUT VITAMIN G?"

## (Quackery, Complementary and Alternative Medicine)

It was my first few months in practice and the sixteen-year-old patient, Becky, was accompanied by her parents who took me aback with the question. I had just finished my training at Duke, felt that I was up to date on the most recent medical knowledge, and I had to confess that I had never heard of vitamin G. It was a test question and Mom and Dad nodded to each other as if confirming their suspicion that I was ignorant of the latest medical breakthroughs.

Mother and daughter were being treated by a "vitaminologist" in Florida. He had Becky taking sixty vitamin pills daily, including his own vitamin G concoction. He said she had hepatitis based on abnormal blood tests, which were actually related to muscle inflammation rather than liver disease. According to him, a rising sedimentation rate was an indicator that the patient was getting better. Wrong. The sedimentation rate is like your golf score, you want it lower not higher. Above all, the parents were told not to let anyone put her on prednisone. The parents agreed with his caveat.

Becky had been referred by Dr. Harold Riley, a local neurologist, who thought she might have a connective tissue disease like lupus or polymyositis (an inflammatory muscle illness). I suspected he was right, but would need a muscle biopsy and special neurologic studies to clarify the diagnosis. Hospital admission was arranged and I started the patient, in spite of reluctance by the parents, on prednisone. Becky and her family were Jehovah's Witnesses and I pictured a worst case scenario of prednisone causing a fatal gastrointestinal bleeding episode in someone who would not accept a transfusion. Would I have one of the shortest practices in the history of Lynchburg medicine?

Fortunately, all went well. Laboratory studies and muscle biopsy reports suggested a condition called Mixed Connective Tissue Disease (MCTD). Dr. Gordon Sharp, an academic medical center rheumatologist, pioneered the recognition of this illness and my patient's studies reflected the mixed elements of inflammatory muscle disease, vasculitis (inflammation of blood vessels) and skin changes like scleroderma.

This responded dramatically to low dose prednisone, and when Becky returned to the office two weeks after hospital discharge, I was gratified to hear that for the first time in two years she felt normal. Symptoms of pain and weakness in muscles and joints had resolved. Chronic fatigue abated. All abnormal blood tests returned to normal, and we gingerly adjusted her prednisone dose to 10 mg every other day with no signs of side effects. The long term outcome for MCTD was unknown. Would some patients develop deforming arthritis, myositis, or scleroderma? With no signs of inflammation, the prognosis seemed excellent.

Then the family moved to North Carolina. I arranged follow up with a Duke rheumatologist who preceded me in training, optimistic she would do well. Several years later, however, I received a consult to see Becky in the hospital. She was admitted for orthopedic hand surgery.

After the family moved away, they did not see the rheumatologist, but instead saw a physician who stopped her prednisone and espoused water therapy and vitamins again. Erosive, deforming arthritis progressed and she eventually evolved into a scleroderma condition with chronic lung and heart problems which would prove fatal. In spite of treatment with strong medicines including cyclophosphamide, methotrexate, and prednisone, we were never able to gain control of her disease as we had initially with low dose prednisone.

Was a young person robbed of her youth and life because of the allure of quackery? Forms of complementary and alternative medicine (CAM) are constantly being tried by our patients. In one study, over 38 percent of patients had used them in the preceding twelve months. This included natural products such as herbal medicines, vitamins, and probiotics; mind-body treatment including meditation, yoga, tai-chi, and hypnosis; manipulative and body-based spinal manipulation and massage therapy; movement therapies (Feldenkrais Method, Pilates, Rolfing); traditional faith healers; energy treatments such as magnets or light treatments; and some whole medical systems such as traditional Chinese medicine.

The NIH (National Institutes of Health) and Georgetown Medical Center have looked at these alternative drug therapies and modalities of treatment from a scientific standpoint. Some of these are found to be helpful, but should not be used to the exclusion of conventional treatment. Publications such as *Arthritis Today, Arthritis Self Management, Arthritis & Rheumatism,* and information from the Arthritis Foundation provide updated reviews of alternative and complementary treatments.

In general, trials of these therapies were assumed to cause no harm. However, in early 2015, many over-the-counter (OTC) vitamin and herb preparations were found to contain none of the touted active ingredients and some contained potentially harmful additives or fillers. The FDA will need to monitor the CAMs just like prescription medications.

I began to understand the attraction of these medicines and treatments early in my career thanks to my Aunt Ruth, the late Mrs. Milton S. Bush of Salem, West Virginia. (See..."I Know What You Doctors Say, But...").

# "THIS HEADACHE IS DIFFERENT"
## (Sometimes It *Is* Brain Surgery)

B. J. had been followed in my office for eight years with fibromyalgia. She was forty-four years old, worked full-time as a bookkeeper, and was raising two children approaching their teenage years. There was plenty of stress juggling the roles of wife, mother, and office worker. She had handled the arthralgias, myalgias, and fatigue of fibromyalgia fairly well with her nonsteroidal etodolac medicine, sleep modification, taking low dose amitriptyline, and aerobic exercise when possible. Her last office visit was six months ago and in the interim she had developed headaches and neck pain. She had seen a neurologist who checked an MRI of the brain, interpreted the MRI as normal, and diagnosed a migraine equivalent headache. Topamax and pain meds weren't helping.

Headaches are not unusual in fibromyalgia patients and, in young to middle-aged females, any new headache is assumed to be a migraine or migraine equivalent, just like any abdominal complaint is diagnosed initially as irritable bowel syndrome. But having taken care of B. J. for some time, I knew it was significant when she felt that this headache was different. Tension headaches are often related to neck pain and I had my x-ray technician take some cervical spine films. Degenerative disc disease was present at several levels, which might relate to neck pain precipitating a tension headache, but the real clue was in the lateral skull film we always included with the C spine. This provides a view of the sella, the part of the brain that encloses the pituitary gland. It should be the size of a dime. B.J.'s sella was larger than a quarter, suggesting a pituitary tumor. I asked the neurologist to review the MRI with attention to that area. He confirmed the presence of the pituitary tumor. She was referred to UVa and was cured with subsequent brain surgery.

When I was a medical student and during my post-graduate internship, internal medicine residency, and rheumatology fellowship, I was taught clinical radiology by Dr. George Baylin. He was a pioneer in Duke radiology and he always stressed obtaining the maximum information from each x-ray. If we ordered a chest x-ray on one of our lupus patients, he recommended that the patient hold the hands just below the ribs to get a look at possible related arthritis changes in addition to lupus related lung or heart problems. When shooting the lateral C spine x-ray, include the lateral skull film with the upper C spine to visualize the sella. Once or twice a year, a patient was found to have an enlarged sella indicating a pituitary tumor. Currently, if x-rays are ordered from radiology, a lateral skull film to check sella size is considered to be a separate x-ray; hand films would never be interpreted on a chest x-ray view; and wrist x-rays are not part of routine hand films. This increases radiation exposure and health care costs.

Before doing x-rays in my own office, I had films done by the hospital or Radiology Consultants. It was an inconvenience for the patients, but I always had them bring the films for my review and to explain the findings to the patient. In the second year of practice (1980), one of our excellent CCU nurses came for an evaluation of arthritis in her hands. This fifty-five-year-old white female had been diagnosed with osteoarthritis and was told nothing could be done for arthritis (fighting words for the rheumatologist). Her medical history included bilateral carpal tunnel surgery within the preceding four or five years. One of the Lynchburg Family Practice residents (Dr. Francis Carter) was taking an elective rotation with me. The patient indeed had bony changes of the distal finger joints (Heberden's nodes) and the proximal interphalangeal joints (Bouchard's nodes) compatible with significant osteoarthritis, but she also had changes in the metacarpophalangeal joints (knuckles at the base of the fingers)—an unusual location for osteoarthritis. (See... "I Don't Drink That Much.") When we reviewed her x-rays, the usual irregular joint space narrowing typical of osteoarthritis was not present; instead joint space was maintained or increased with bony spur changes about all the joints. When we reviewed her cervical spine films, a fifty-cent-piece-size sella suggested a pituitary tumor. Acromegaly was diagnosed ultimately and successful transsphenoidal resection carried out. The official interpretation by radiology was osteoarthritis and there was no mention of the enlarged sella. Knowing the clinical history and clues such as a history of carpal tunnel surgery, unusual pattern in distribution of joint involvement, and increasing joint space allowed a more specific evaluation of the x-rays. The patient later brought in a driver's license picture from five years earlier showing facial changes of acromegaly that had evolved gradually.

Sometimes a new patient would seem aggravated with the comprehensive initial history and physical exam. Frequently, the patient had excellent care by his primary care doctor and he was impatient, just here for some arthritis treatment. One such patient was J. B., a sixty-eight year old white male with a two-year history of diabetes followed by Dr. Charles Sackett, one of our finest internists. There was no family history of diabetes. J. B. was referred for evaluation of hand pain which persisted after carpal tunnel surgery. In addition, he was having visual problems attributed, like the carpal tunnel, to his diabetes.

There can be several rheumatologic manifestations related to diabetes, but usually with longer standing disease. He had mild osteoarthritis hand changes. In going through the review of systems, he had noted worsening vision with decreased peripheral vision looking straight ahead, and a change in his dental bite. The recent onset of diabetes, the history of carpal tunnel syndrome and visual changes, prompted a look at his sella. An MRI showed a pituitary tumor beginning to impinge on an area, called the optic chiasm, was causing his visual changes. Neurosurgery was performed as quickly as possible, his vision was preserved, and acromegaly was diagnosed.

I always felt that to be a good subspecialist (rheumatologist), you needed to be a good specialist (internist). In this day of subspecialization, it is easy to narrow your focus in evaluating the patient. The electronic medical record review of systems emphasizes what's not present and hinders investigation of pertinent negatives or areas outside the particular problem at that visit. While some patients and physicians may feel that "it's just arthritis, it's not brain surgery," sometimes they're wrong and as these patients found, it *is* brain surgery. You won't find out if you don't consider the possibility, and you see what you know.

# "YOU SAVED MY LIFE—TWICE"

I was seeing C. W. in follow-up after a recent hospitalization. The lifesaving he alluded to was not a dramatic cardiopulmonary resuscitation (CPR) after cardiac arrest nor a Heimlich maneuver to relieve a blocked airway.

The first incident related to a routine part of patient history called the review of systems (ROS). Often in the haste of shortened office visit time, the ROS may simply be noted as "noncontributory," usually meaning it wasn't done. Sometimes a problem specific ROS may be obtained. For following rheumatoid arthritis, attention may be directed more to morning stiffness, new or worsening joint involvement, signs of medication intolerance—any skin rash or stomach upset. But I usually asked, "Anything new going on with your health? Any chest pain, belly pain, shortness of breath or stomach upset?" C. W.'s response? "Nah, Doc, just some heartburn."

I had been taking care of C. W.'s rheumatoid arthritis over the past ten years. This seventy-six-year-old was active, rode a motorcycle, lifted weights, and hunted. He was a non-complaining stoic individual. His RA was doing well. I needed to know more about this heartburn. How long had this been going on? Any reflux with it? Any relation to food? What brings it on? What relieves it?

The heartburn had been present for only two to three weeks. There was no reflux, and he couldn't relate it to any particular foods. It seemed to come on with physical activity, was relieved with rest, and he noted no difference taking a swig of antacid. A popular television commercial at that time portrayed a patient who thought he had heart problems but it was all due to reflux—"My doctor said Mylanta." I pointed out to C. W., as I did to all my patients, that "My doctor says Mylanta" is fine but *only* after you rule out heart disease.

I referred C. W. to cardiology and started the patient on a daily baby aspirin while awaiting their evaluation. As soon as the cardiologist saw C. W., an urgent cardiac catheterization was arranged with placement of three stents in his coronary arteries. Heartburn was gone and a possible heart attack was averted.

The second time I saved C. W.'s life was likewise not dramatic. He had been hospitalized with a fever of unknown origin (FUO). He was on the hospitalist service (his primary care physician, like most now, did not have hospital admitting privileges) and an occult infection was suspected. Infection is the most common cause of an FUO followed by cancers and then rheumatologic diseases. I was notified of his admission for a courtesy consult, his wife having requested this.

C. W. looked terrible. In the weeks preceding the hospitalization, his primary physician had treated him with doxycycline for suspected Lyme disease followed by a course of Bactrim or Septra (trimethoprim sulfamethoxazole—TMP/SMX)—one of the few antibiotics to be avoided by any patient, like C.W., on methotrexate for rheumatoid arthritis. Daily fever spikes to 102 degrees were accompanied by diffuse red rash, severe arthralgias in all his joints, and a confused mental state. I suspected he was having a drug reaction to the antibiotics and recommended discontinuing all antibiotics and beginning intravenous steroids. His condition improved quickly and C. W. was discharged on tapering doses of prednisone. Not dramatic to some, but, more importantly, lifesaving to C. W.

There is some advantage to long term continuity of care for our patients. This is lost in the hospitalist system in which the patient's primary physician, who should know the medical history best, is not directing the care. Even in the hospital, care is fragmented as the patient may be seen by several hospitalists during the admission. More frequent transitions of care are associated with more chances for errors.

With the time compression the primary physician experiences related to documentation requirements of the EMR (Electronic Medical Record), there is a tendency for acute problems to be directed by the primary doctor to an urgent care facility or the hospital ER. Less efficient care by physicians, PAs (physician assistants), or NPs (nurse practitioners) who don't know the patient usually results in greater health care costs.

It was suggested by a retired hospital administrator and medical ethicist that this new system of fragmented care is expected by our patients and my reticence relates to my age. But that's not what I hear from patients, and it's their lives we want to save—sometimes twice.

# "I've Got the Gouch"

## (Gout—It's Not a Bowl of Cherries—Or Is It?)

My patient didn't know it, but he expressed the clinical problem of acute gout very well. The degree of pain is reported to be second only to childbirth and passing a kidney stone. "G-Ouch," indeed. Musical allusion might be—"Gout! You Know You Make Me Want to Shout!" And yet, if the rheumatologist had to have one of the conditions he treats, he would choose gout—with the proviso that he could tolerate medicines like colchicine and allopurinol.

The definitive textbook on gout (*Gout and Hyperuricemia*) was written by Dr. James B. Wyngaarden and Dr. William Kelley during the time I was at Duke. All metabolic pathways and every enzyme involved in gout are known. Studies carried out on the research ward included having patients on a purine restricted diet for several weeks. Excluded were foods high in purine, which included sweetbreads. As a transplanted Yankee, I assumed, as I bet you did, that sweetbreads meant donuts, bear claws, and Danish pastries. Wrong. Sweetbreads refer to animal organ meat. But who eats pancreas, kidney, liver, brains, etc.? A few brave souls eat liver and my wife's relatives in Scotland partake of haggis, the ultimate sweetbread—a pudding made up of heart, liver, and lungs, usually from a sheep, made into a gruel of suet, onions, and oatmeal, served in the stomach of the animal. No wonder there are so few Scottish cookbooks. But who knows what's in our sausage, hot dogs, and processed meats? In any event, after two weeks of such a restricted diet on the research unit, the patient's blood level of uric acid usually came down only one or two points. Normal uric acid levels run from 2.3 to 6.6 mg/dl, while many of our research subjects had levels of 11 or 12. My take away message was that the inherited metabolic pathways for uric acid were more important than diet.

Once in practice, however, I continued to have patients relate a flare of their gout after eating different foods. "Doc, if I eat (pick one or more: shrimp, pinto beans, hot dogs, country ham, liver, pork, beef) my gout flares up." I assured them that on the basis of our marvelous advanced science, this was probably all in their heads. And I was wrong. I learned my lesson about diet and gout from the late Dr. Frank Whitehouse, one of our most distinguished silver-haired retired physicians. Frank was an avid outdoorsman, marksman, and bird hunter. He was elected president of the local chitlin society and presented to my office several days after their fall festival with an acute attack of podagra (classic gout attacking the large toe). There is nothing more sweetbread than chitlins (hog intestines prepared as food). My needle barely touched his exquisitely tender, red, swollen large toe when out poured a stream of white liquid—this looks like pus, but under a special polarized microscope it is a mass of uric acid crystals (milk of urate). Lesson learned. I now ask my patients if they relate any foods to a flare of their gout; if so, avoid that food. But as one patient said, "Sometimes you just have to have a hotdog." I know what you mean. (See… "I Don't Deserve The Best. What's Second Best?")

I learned early in training when angry or upset to swallow my smoke, but one patient's wife pushed me to the limit. My eighty-two-year-old patient had suffered with gout for forty years, developing deforming arthritis with large deposits of gout (tophi) around elbows, knees and fingers. The minute I entered the exam room, before the patient or I could speak, his wife demanded, "Tell him about cherries for gout." I explained that while we had heard about cherries and gout for years, there really was no good evidence of its benefit. I then proceeded with his history and physical examination and left the room to begin completing the EMR entries before returning with written information on gout and explaining how we needed to treat his gout.

However, the minute I re-entered the exam room, the wife accosted me once more. "No, really, tell him about cherries." By this time, I was peeved and irritated. I was close to telling her that cherries for gout was an old wives' tale, and she was an old wife. I swallowed the smoke and held my tongue, but let her see my irritation and proceeded with educating and treating the patient.

For years, I reassured my gout patients that we would be able to control their illness with inexpensive medicines. Flare-ups of acute gout could be controlled with colchicine; long term control achieved with allopurinol. We had over fifty years of experience with these meds. Colchicine was made by several companies and cost less than a penny per pill—until the government got involved. Colchicine was developed before the FDA existed. In their wisdom, the FDA decided that colchicine needed to be put through similar trials required for new meds. One company (Takeda) did this, and we found out nothing we had not learned with the use of colchicine over decades. But the FDA had created a monopoly and the price rose to over $5.00 a pill. An editorial in *Journal of the American Medical Association* (Guglielmo, B.J., "The Colchicine Debacle," 2/11/14, 184) discussed this. My gout patients substituted inexpensive prednisone in place of the new, expensive colchicine, but we began to worry that the FDA might decide that prednisone and allopurinol needed FDA approval. Hopefully not.

Expecting the standard meds would take care of my patient's gout, I dismissed the question of adding cherries to the regimen. Wrong again. In over forty years as a physician, I have learned that nothing is set in stone. So there was only mild surprise when two weeks after this encounter, an article appeared in our major rheumatology journal (*Arthritis & Rheumatism;* Y. Zhang, et al., "Cherry Consumption and Decreased Risk of Recurrent Gout Attacks" Vol. 64; Dec 2012) and, guess what? Cherries *are* good for gout. I continue to be humbled and educated by our patients and their families. An old wives' tale has become part of an old rheumatologist's treatment regimen. However, we still need our advanced scientific knowledge and medicines like allopurinol and colchicine because gout treatment is not *just* a bowl of cherries.

# "I DON'T DESERVE THE BEST. WHAT'S SECOND BEST?"

## (About Gout)

This was a surprising statement from easily the most affluent patient cared for in my practice. I doubt that L. T. ever travelled in less than first class accommodations; he was my only patient chauffeured to his appointments. Now retired, his life on a magnificent estate in Virginia horse country was filled with "women, wine, and song" as the saying goes. Overweight, hypertensive, and diabetic, he resisted his family physician's efforts to restrict calories, alcohol, salt, and rich foods in his diet. And that's where I came into the picture. He had gout. He was a prototype for the image of the rich land owner sitting with his swollen red foot elevated—excruciating pain so severe he couldn't stand the weight of a sheet touching it.

Frankly, his care exasperated me. For several years, I could count on seeing him after every major holiday: the Fourth of July, Labor Day, Thanksgiving, Christmas, and New Year's. Dietary and alcohol excesses were the culprits inciting a flare of his gout time after time.

Based on sound scientific knowledge, (See…"I've Got the Gouch"), with attention to certain dietary restrictions and the use of inexpensive medicines like prednisone and allopurinol, the disease could be controlled and flare-ups prevented. That is, *if* the patient would comply.

For the umpteenth time, after yet another post-Thanksgiving gouty flare, I was simultaneously instructing and berating my patient. "L. T., the best thing you can do to take care of your gout is avoid these rich foods, eliminate all forms of alcohol, and take your meds." He considered the advice briefly and responded, "You know, Doc, I've abused my body so much over all these years that I don't deserve the best. What's second best?"

Discussion of a diet low in purines and sweetbreads (animal organ derived meats) and restriction of alcohol would fall on deaf ears. He wasn't about to exchange his life style of "women, wine, and song" for, as they said in the early 1960s, "Metracal, the same old gal, and sing along with Mitch." Better just give him a cortisone injection and keep an appointment space open after Christmas.

# "ONE OF YOUR PATIENTS PRAYED FOR YOU"

What an honor. After Sunday school one day, Betty Jo Hamner, a pillar of our First Pres (First Presbyterian Church) family, shared this kind news with me. At a weekly meeting of her prayer group, my patient, Laurie Babcock, offered a prayer for me. She was not only a patient, but a personal friend seriously ill with scleroderma. Progressive pulmonary disease complicating her illness left her severely short of breath with any exertion. Yet she prayed for me.

For several years we provided a spirituality and health ministry message at the office. My staff (See…"You Have the Best Office") helped develop this handout for our patients:

## SPIRITUALITY, RELIGION, AND HEALTH

In March 2001, my wife and I attended a conference at Duke titled "Faith in the Future." The speakers first introduced us to the problem of health care costs rapidly rising out of control in spite of health insurance companies attempting to rein in health expenditures by restricting care and services. Aging baby boomers promised to overwhelm the system.

The first hospitals and institutions for medical care were formed by churches. Could religion and spirituality in today's high tech environment play a role in controlling costs? The director of the conference, Dr. Harold Koenig of Duke, suggests that they could. In his book, *Handbook of Religion and Health,* he cites over 2,000 studies showing the health benefits of attendance and involvement in church or synagogue and practices such as intercessory prayer.

During the past twenty (now thirty-five) years of medical practice, I have been impressed by the impact of faith in a

patient's ability to cope with illness and respond to treatment. While we encourage our patients to be involved in
a formal faith community, we would like to include our
patients in daily intercessory prayer.

This is Dr. Wilson's prayer for his patients:

Heavenly Father, be especially close to all our patients.
Heal those who may be healed so they may not need our
help. Comfort all and decrease the pain and inflammation
they suffer. May the medicines work to our patients' benefit without bothersome side effects. Grant us the wisdom
to provide the best care for our patients.

The staff of the Lynchburg Rheumatology Clinic would like
to include you in our prayer. Let us know if this is acceptable to you with respect to your faith and beliefs.

Jeffrey W. Wilson, M.D.

Laurie's prayer might have appropriately asked God for
more wisdom and direction for her physician, but I suspect the
prayer recognized the concern and distress we shared regarding
her declining health and acknowledged all of us being part of
God's plan. Her favorite Psalm was 121:

"I lift up my eyes to the hills.
From whence does my help come?
My help comes from the Lord,
who made heaven and earth.

He will not let your foot be moved,
he who keeps you will not slumber.
Behold, he who keeps Israel
will neither slumber nor sleep.

The Lord is your keeper;
the Lord is your shade on your right hand.
The sun shall not smite you by day,
nor the moon by night.

The Lord will keep you from all evil;
he will keep your life.
The Lord will keep
Your going out and your coming in
From this time forth and for evermore. (RSV)

She recognized, and I believe was reassured, that God was in control.

There was only one patient who openly objected to our prayer. Ironically, he had been raised as a true Southern Baptist with church every Sunday and Wednesday prayer meeting each week. When I met him, he was reading *The Atheist's Bible* for a second time. He suggested that from an intellectual point of view, one could not accept conventional religion. About that time I read Francis Collins's wonderful book, *The Language of God*. Dr. Collins is a renowned scientist who supervised the Human Genome Project and became director of the National Institutes of Health. It not only portrays the story of Dr. Collins's journey from atheist to believer, but also outlines the science versus religion arguments contesting atheism with more scholarship and clarity than I possess. I sent my patient a Christmas card that year recommending the book to him. No response. You do what you can.

The majority of patients welcomed the letter and prayers. Many included our office in their prayers, and extended personal prayers later for my wife's breast cancer treatment and my Parkinson's disease. Prayer begets prayer. One patient, during his office visit, even combined a prayer for my scheduled spinal stenosis back surgery with a laying on of hands to the area of pain. How kind and thoughtful.

We kept a Bible in each exam room and as I entered the room, my patient often would be reading a passage. This always opened up a brief discussion of chapter and verse or Sunday school studies. While there was no code nor documentation criteria to put a monetary number on this interaction, it certainly was valuable and enriched the patient-physician relationship.

A book by William Diehl, *The Monday Connection,* discusses the problem of continuing your faith and religious principles beyond Sunday and into your day-to-day work. A health ministry in a medical office seemed like a natural fit. Maybe it would not work in other places, but the majority of our Central Virginia patients have a strong faith. Many of their churches have healing services. I attended several evening healing services at Quaker Presbyterian and was impressed with the impact of the service on patients, family members, and health care workers.

Our First Presbyterian Church started a prayer committee. As a member, I learned a great deal about prayer from our associate minister, Walter Smith. While we may pray for healing, we recognize that it may not be part of God's plan. We always pray for the Heavenly Father to be close to the patient. May the patient feel His eternal love and presence and feel comforted by that. A physician providing voluntary care at Mother Teresa's mission in India asked her advice in working with the patients. He was told, "Don't ever let them feel they're alone—because they're not. God is always with them."

I am sure Laurie felt this. I will always remember being paged urgently to Lynchburg General the afternoon she died (February 7, 2005). I rushed to the hospital and met her sister, Meg Laughon, in the parking lot. Laurie had just passed away in the CCU (Cardiac Care Unit). We cried together. Maybe she was at first surprised to see my emotional response, but Meg understood and said, "You loved her, too, didn't you?" Of course. Meg remembers a rainbow appearing as she drove home that evening—a sign to her that Laurie was being welcomed into God's heavenly kingdom.

Perhaps some physicians consider it unprofessional or unmanly to cry for patients. It has been part of the total patient experience for me as their physician. I've cried for joy with healing of disease, cried in sadness with deaths of patients, and cried with many as we said goodbye when closing the office. Remember Coach Jim Valvano's advice when he delivered his memorable speech at the ESPYs: "Every day think, laugh, and cry." It makes a full day. Over the thirty-five years, my patients provided the opportunity to share all three with them. It enhanced and fulfilled our practice.

Since retiring December 15, 2014, I still pray for my patients with a modified daily prayer. "Heavenly Father, be close to all my patients: past, present, and future (I see new rheumatology patients in the Free Clinic). Heal those who may be healed so they may not need medical care. Ease the pain and inflammation in all our patients. May their medicines be effective and well tolerated with no bad side effects. Grant to me and their other physicians wisdom in caring for and learning to care about our patients."

Imagine improving our health with treatments that cost nothing and have no bad side effects: religion, spirituality and prayer. Now that's good medicine.

# "AREN'T I DISABLED NOW?"
## (Antiphospholipid Antibody Syndrome)

I was called to the Emergency Room to see a patient with arthritis. The fifty-eight-year-old African American female had inflammatory arthritis of her hands and a family history of a sister with lupus. Review of old hospital records revealed a brief hospitalization earlier that year (1985) with thrombophlebitis (blood clot) in her right leg. Could these be related? We were just beginning to appreciate hypercoagulable (increased tendency for blood to clot) problems in patients with connective tissue disorders like lupus. While the patient did not meet diagnostic criteria for lupus, the possibility of an antiphospholipid antibody syndrome (APLAS), was confirmed with elevated levels of antibodies on blood tests.

This was my first patient diagnosed with this condition, and I was excited. These hypercoagulability disorders could present with blood clots anywhere in venous or arterial systems, causing phlebitis in the extremities, life threatening clots in lungs (pulmonary emboli) or strokes from thrombosis in the brain. The excitement related to picking up a condition which could be treated with an inexpensive blood thinner medication, Coumadin, and preventing these potentially serious complications. We were just beginning to realize that these patients would have to be on chronic, life-long anticoagulation with blood thinned significantly as indicated by Protime testing (goal of INR 3 to 3.5). The inconvenience of daily Coumadin therapy and frequent monitoring of blood tests was well worth the benefit. The patient was discharged from the hospital on 5 mg Coumadin daily–a fairly significant dose.

Return visit to the office in two weeks showed inadequate anticoagulation and the dose was increased to 7.5 mg daily. Follow up visits were always the same. At each visit, we had to boost up the dose of Coumadin until she was on 15 mg daily, and each time she asked the same question, "Aren't I disabled now? Shouldn't I be getting disability?" I stressed the importance of diagnosing this condition before a disabling complication occurred. We were lucky to have this opportunity. But, I was perplexed with inadequate anticoagulation in spite of increasing doses of Coumadin. My primary care and cardiology friends follow more patients on Coumadin, especially for conditions like atrial fibrillation. They did not seem to have such problems thinning the blood, but this condition was different and I assumed these larger doses were necessary. The patient said she was taking the medicine correctly.

After following the patient over the next four months, I was called again to the ER. She presented with a severe stroke paralyzing the right side of her body associated with slurred speech and expressive aphasia. History from the family revealed that she had not been taking her Coumadin. Her recurrent question was answered. "Yes, now you're disabled." Frankly, I was more depressed than angry. We had diagnosed a new condition treatable with inexpensive medicine which the patient did not take. I couldn't help but recall patients with conditions we could not control who would have gladly complied with such a simple treatment. An opportunity lost.

Over thirty-five years of practice, I have encountered more patients like Eugene Morris. (See..."You're The Doc.") Eugene had severe, long standing inflammatory arthritis–probably an overlapping rheumatoid arthritis and spondyloarthropathy. In spite of multiple surgeries related to his active arthritis, his spirit and attitude helped him complete a career in Forestry and Land management while doing cattle farming on the side. He, like many of my patients, would have qualified for disability, but he resisted and maintained his independent character. He would not be disabled mentally or physically.

The problem of disability in our current society was discussed in an article by Jonah Goldberg (editor at large, *National Review Online*). "Are disability payments the new welfare?" The British government wanted to have their disability recipients

undergo medical testing to determine if they were still too disabled to work. A third of the recipients (878,000) dropped out
of the program, never showing up for testing. Of those retested,
55 percent were found able to work. In our country, changes
over the past fifty years are notable. In 1960, 0.65 percent of
our work force were receiving Social Security disability insurance payments (134 people were working for every officially
recognized disabled worker). Over the last fifty years, there has
been a nine-fold increase to 5.6 percent receiving disability,
with sixteen people working per every disabled worker.

The legal profession has prospered by representing the disability recipient. The lawyers get a cut of every winning recipient's "back pay." Hence, ads on TV, "Disabled? Get the money
you deserve!" Disability programs, Mr. Goldberg points out, are
sometimes taking the place of welfare for those who feel locked
out of the workforce. State governments benefit as states pay
for welfare, but the federal government pays for disabilities. Of
course, you and I, as taxpayers, pay at either level.

While we clearly need a system to help disabled individuals, we should verify their continuing disabled status. Periodic
retesting seems prudent as suggested by the experience in Brit-
ain.

# "I KNOW WHAT'S WRONG"

## (Lupus and Age)

Good thing the patient knew what was wrong because the ER doctor, Walter Beverly, and I weren't sure. I had taken care of W. S. for three years. He was eighty-seven years old when first seen in consultation with problems of fever, anemia, arthralgias, and shortness of breath, possibly related to pleural effusion (fluid around his lungs). Lab tests confirmed a diagnosis of lupus and, like most patients presenting as lupus in the elderly, he responded to low dose prednisone and hydroxychloroquine (Plaquenil). He remained asymptomatic for years on his medical regimen, but now came to the ER with fever, malaise, and shortness of breath.

When the lupus patient is acutely ill, the doctor often finds himself clinically between a rock and a hard place. Is the patient's primary disease—his lupus—more active, causing the symptoms and indicating the need for higher doses of steroids acutely or is a different problem, such as infection, behind his worsened condition? If infection was present, would the steroids make him more susceptible to infection and was there a case for reducing steroids? In some patients, an acute illness might cause a systemic inflammatory response with more active lupus and he might require more steroids while treating for a suspected infection.

Blood studies and x-rays had been obtained. Walter and I stood at the patient's bedside reviewing test results, puzzling over the different diagnoses. My ninety-year-old patient, perhaps sensing our conundrum, offered his analysis. "I know what's wrong—I got too much age on me."

He was a least partly right. Age plays a role in acute and chronic illnesses. As we get older, we have less reserve for fighting diseases like pneumonia. Acute illnesses always stress the reserve but present no problem until a critical illness level is met. As depicted in this schematic, at older age an illness that was tolerated a decade before now puts the patient in this critical disease state. What our systems tolerated and overcame at age forty may be fatal at age eighty. A similar episodic illness does not reach a critical level of illness at 40, 50 or 60 years of age in spite of diminishing reserve until that level of critical illness is reached at 70 years of age and beyond.

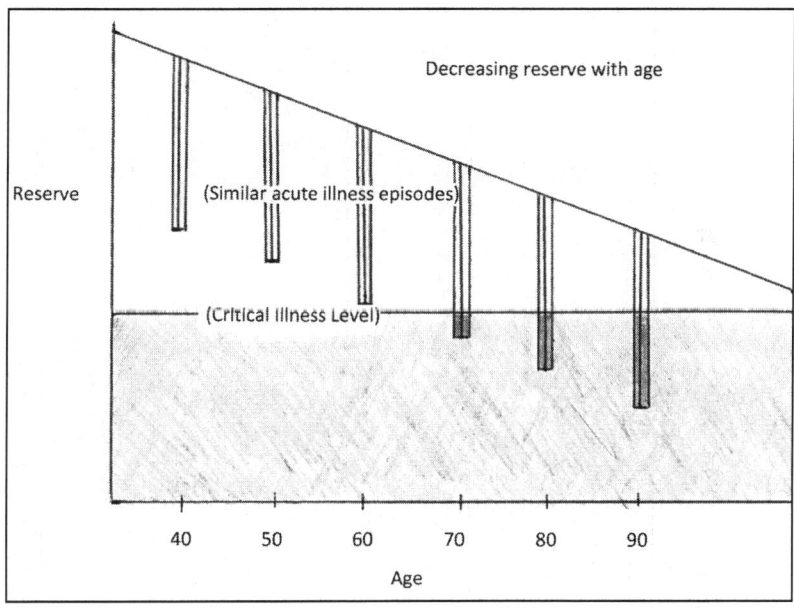

Sometimes it's difficult for patients and families to understand the fragile nature associated with the age-related lack of reserve. Several years ago I was called to see M.B., a ninety-three-year-old man on the psychiatry unit. His astute psychiatrist realized that the altered mental status was due to pneumonia rather than psychiatric illness. I transferred M. B. to a medical ward. The patient lived in Virginia Beach and was visiting his sons in Lynchburg. The family noted that only a year before he was mentally sharp and physically fit enough to go sailing in the ocean with his seventy-plus-year-old sons. What happened? He had enjoyed great health but the pneumonia overwhelmed his age-related diminished reserve, leaving him critically ill. Over the next several weeks improvement in the pneumonia initially was complicated by aspiration, lung and heart failure, and kidney shutdown. The patient did not survive. At age fifty or sixty he probably would have had successful outpatient oral antibiotic treatment of his pneumonia with no comorbid effects on mental status or vital organ function. Age was the difference.

Since becoming Medicare eligible as one of the first baby boomers, I blame less and less on age. In fact, rather than "age related," I often use the term "maturity onset," probably a form of denial. Besides, infomercials notwithstanding, you can't do much about age. I am reminded of an episode of "Sanford and Sons" where Fred delivered a biting retort to his sister-in-law's comment that when she was born, she was blessed by Mother Nature. "Yeah, and after that you were cursed by Father Time."

Eventually, like my patient, W. S., we all will have "too much age" on us. It's just a matter of time.

# "YOU'RE RETIRING ON ME—AGAIN?"

During the last six months of my practice (July to December 2014), patients asked two questions frequently. "You're retiring on me again?" and "Are you glad you came back?" The first question was addressed by reminding them that neither retirement was of my choosing. Economic factors forced the closing of the Lynchburg Rheumatology Clinic in 2010 (See "...I Can't See How You Can Stay in Practice") while health and economic factors played a role in ending Rheumatology of CVFP.

The second question was easy to answer. I will always be glad I came back. It allowed me to extend some long-term relationships with patients I cared for and cared about over the past thirty plus years. A parting note to our patients summarized our feelings. It had been a privilege and honor to serve them, and while I would not be there to care *for* them (provide medical services), I would still care *about* them. And I do.

When I consider some things I would have missed, I am even more grateful to have had the additional three-and-a-half years of practice. Some extraordinary cases presented which I had not seen before. A middle-aged (fifty-plus years old) woman was referred by the excellent Nurse Practitioner, Joe Davis, at Charlotte Court House with biopsy proven small vessel inflammation (vasculitis) which was induced by chronic minocycline treatment for adult acne and associated with a special blood test (P-ANCA). This resolved with a prednisone taper and discontinuing the minocycline. The sister of my former office manager, Sharon Sirocco, presented with cryoglobulinemic vasculitis (an inflammation of blood vessels with a protein which caused special problems in cooler fingers and toes) as the initial manifestation of multiple myeloma associated with hypercalcemia (elevated blood calcium levels). A younger male was diagnosed with vitamin C deficiency, mimicking vasculitis and angioedema related to alpha gal tick disease.

After I returned to practice in July 2011, Dr. Frank Sauls-bury, the only pediatric rheumatologist at UVa, retired with no immediate replacement. We assumed care for his patients from our locale and saw new juvenile rheumatology patients as well. One case of rheumatic fever was diagnosed in a young girl, and a teenage male patient with Familial Mediterranean Fever was followed for treatment with a biologic agent under the guidance of the Cleveland Clinic.

Two female patients (one mid-forties and the other early fifties) were diagnosed with overlapping connective tissue disease and multiple sclerosis. One of them was referred to me soon after I returned to practice with a question of retinal vasculitis (inflammation of blood vessels in the back part of the eye), possibly related to sarcoidosis. Concerns about CNS (Central Nervous System [brain and spinal cord]) vasculitis prompted evaluation and follow-up at Johns Hopkins with the diagnosis of MS established only shortly before my practice ended. The patient, her sister, and mother are HLA B27 positive. (See... "Your Father Took Care of My Mother.") The other patient had polymyositis (inflammatory muscle condition) overlapping with her MS.

Of special interest was investigation of alpha gal tick disease. (See..."My Doctor Thinks I Have Lupus.") During the last fifteen months of practice, I checked over 200 patients for possible tick-related disease. One patient had definite Lyme disease; one patient had Ehrlichiosis; one had Rocky Mountain Spotted Fever; and 147 tested positive for alpha gal tick disease. Like Lyme disease, while most of my patients presented with musculoskeletal symptoms, there were protean manifestations. Twelve of 147 had skin problems, including urticarial vasculitis, perivascular dermatitis, serpiginous urticarial rash, nummular eczema, and subcutaneous nodules. Several patients had diarrhea after beef exposure and some patients noted improvement in IBS (Irritable Bowel Syndrome) symptoms with diet restriction, and several noted less abdominal pain, which previously occurred regularly four to five hours after mammalian meat ingestion. One patient had improvement in paresthesias (numb-

84

ness and tingling of fingers and toes). Twenty-eight of the 147 patients were referred for evaluation of a (+) ANA test. These were felt to be false (+) tests as part of their alpha gal tick disease without diagnostic criteria met for lupus. Two of the patients are neighbors sharing the same population of ticks.

In conversation with the lab director for Viracor-IBT, where the tests are run, it's not felt that the alpha gal test is a sensitive test with a lot of false positive results. The levels of the test did not seem to correlate with different clinical manifestations nor severity of symptoms. One family had father and son with levels >100 kU/L. They are cattle ranchers with no obvious mammalian meat allergy, but had improvement in arthritic and gastrointestinal symptoms after restricting their diet. The test looks for elevated levels of IgE antibodies to galactose-alpha-1, 3 galactose. This test is not part of the routine tick panel of tests and should be added when the physician is considering tick-related diseases.

A fascinating article in March 2008 *New England Journal of Medicine* describes anaphylaxis induced by a biologic agent (cetuximab) for colorectal cancer and squamous cell cancer of the head and neck, appearing mainly in patients in the Southeast. The patients were found to be alpha gal (+), and the reason the reaction occurred more in the Southeast? That's where the ticks are! Of greater importance, as we use more and more biologic agents in virtually all fields of medicine, should this test be checked to forewarn possible anaphylactic reaction to these medicines? Since my retirement, I'm not sure my fellow physicians have followed up on this.

While I continue to miss my patients and interesting new cases, I do not miss the EMR (electronic medical record) one minute. I had the PenChart EMR at the first office and Allscripts (read Oddscripts) at my last office. Someone asked me about my training for the two systems. The most important training occurred over fifty years ago in the ninth grade when my mother made me take typing. By the time I stopped practice, I was essentially typing all day, unable to afford a scribe. I left practice with an appreciation of the intent of EMR, but frustration with its unrealized touted improvements in efficient patient care and quality of care. As one critic notes, it mistakes quantity for quality, and meaningful use with each new tier becomes more meaningless. For example, I was noted to have met meaningful use criteria for childhood asthma—yet never saw a patient with childhood asthma. I probably met meaningful use for brain surgery as well. See the note on "...I don't like that electric record." The EMR and Medicare rules intrude on and weaken the patient-physician relationship. Although I am a Medicare patient, I would understand if, in the future, doctors opt out of Medicare.

# "I WANTED TO FIND OUT
IF YOU KNEW ANYTHING"

Each spring during the first few years of practice, our local Arthritis Foundation support group sponsored a free public
symposium covering varied topics, such as rheumatoid arthritis, lupus, gout, joint replacements, PT, OT and osteoarthritis.
I invited speakers from the rheumatology departments at UVa,
MCV, and Duke. Presentations were scheduled at specific advertised times so an individual could plan to attend the talk
of his or her particular interest. I arranged speakers and topics
while the secretary for the group secured the venue, usually a
room provided free at River Ridge Mall.

At one of the meetings, I noticed my patient T. F. This twen-
ty-eight-year-old white female had a form of arthritis called Reiter's Syndrome (See..."Your Father Took Care of My Mother.")
She was intelligent, industrious, and feisty. "What are you doing here, T? You already know all this stuff." "Yeah," she answered," but I wanted to find out if *you* knew anything." She
was kidding—I think, but it never hurts to get a second opinion,
especially from a medical center, especially free.

I was blessed to have some excellent volunteer secretaries for the Arthritis Support group until it dissolved locally (it
has continued in Roanoke). The secretaries worked for free and
were industrious and enterprising. Prior to starting my practice
in Lynchburg, Dr. William Massie (See..."I Can't Believe You're
Moving to That Stagnant Little Virginia Town") started a monthly free rheumatology clinic at Virginia Baptist Hospital (VBH)
Out Patient Department in which a difficult or challenging case
would be presented to one of the UVa visiting rheumatologists.
Very often, Dr. John Davis, chairman of the rheumatology division, or Dr. Carolyn Brunner, was the attending physician. A patient could not have more erudite and kind doctors evaluating

them. It was free and provided care suggestions for the patient and an excellent learning experience for Dr. Massie and me.

The support group maintained a phone number allowing patients to contact the secretary who would act as a resource for arthritis information, providing brochures, contact numbers to the national Arthritis Foundation, or physician referral. One of our secretaries, Barbara Johnson, arranged a local television broadcast with open phone lines to call-in questions for the rheumatologist. As I sat there, one disgruntled individual called in this query. "I want to know when I called the secretary, why did she refer me to Dr. Wilson for an expensive evaluation instead of to the free rheumatology clinic at VBH?" I looked over at Barbara and said, "You'd better take this one." Incidentally, this was in the early 1980s and my new patient evaluation was $45 and follow-up visit was $15, but it wasn't free.

Medical Center input can be very helpful. Complex patients could have their cases reviewed and at times, weekly conferences would allow the patient's case to be evaluated by several members of the rheumatology division. Sometimes a patient or family member would want a second opinion or were not happy with my care. Two mentoring physicians early in my career—Dr. Richard Hawkins and Dr. George Craddock—gave me the correct perspective. The only way you could lose was by discouraging referral or second opinion. Don't let hubris breed ideas that no one could know more than you, that you are doing everything that can be done, and the patient is wasting his time and money questioning your care. Instead, encourage second opinions, especially by the medical center. Usually the patient came back reassured that they were receiving the right care. Often there was new information for the physician which benefited his patient.

Sometimes, however, even the medical center did not have all the answers. There is increasing interest in complementary or alternative therapy. Acupuncture, chiropractic, yoga, pilates, aroma therapy, naturopathy, integrative medicine may all be helpful for some patients. The NIH and most medical centers are evaluating the merits of these varied treatments. While a student and house officer (intern, resident, fellow) at Duke, I learned a valuable lesson from Dr. Mike McLeod. He was in the gastroenterology division and we considered him a "doctor's doctor." If any of us had a personal internal medicine or GI problem, we would welcome his input in our care. He showed me that you couldn't be a good subspecialist (such as rheumatologist or gastroenterologist) if you weren't a good specialist (internal medicine physician).

Dr. McLeod had patients referred from the entire Southeast—many patients referred with unexplained abdominal pain—the "black box," we called it. The typical Duke GI work-up during a week hospitalization included rigid sigmoidoscopy (flexible scopes were not available then), barium enema, upper gastrointestinal series with small bowel follow-through and a host of blood tests. Many times the work-up was negative and often the patient was felt to have "functional abdominal pain." No clear medical cause was found. Usually the patient returned two weeks after discharge for a final evaluation and review of tests and x-ray results. In one case, several weeks after a patient's return appointment and explanation of no organic cause found for the symptoms, Dr. McLeod received a note. After that expensive work-up at Duke, she had gone to a chiropractor who got rid of her pain with one treatment. "Why didn't you send me to the chiropractor when the Duke work-up was negative?" Lesson learned. After that, Dr. McLeod was praised by patients. "After your thorough negative work-up ruled out serious disease, you were smart enough to refer me to a chiropractor. Thank you."

In today's medical environment, there is a tendency to conclude the patient's care with the comment—"I don't know what you have, but it's not in my field. Goodbye." Sometimes the patient has seen multiple specialists and the suggestion of complementary or alternative therapy gives hope and often significant benefit. It's part of our distinction between caring "for" patients—i.e. providing a medical service and caring "about" patients. Dismissing the patient because the symptoms aren't in your field, without future plans, is incomplete care. Sir William

Osler, one of the godfathers of medicine said, "One thing is certain: it is not for you to don the black cap and...take hope away from any patient...hope that comes to us all." If I can't help you or find out what's causing your symptoms in my field, let's see if we can get help for you from the medical center, by referral to a physician in another field, or trying alternative therapy.

Reevaluation by your physician after a period of time can be helpful as well. Dr. Eugene Stead, past chairman of the department of medicine at Duke, made the point that when the patient went from the basement to the first floor with his doctor, upon arrival at the first floor, the doctor had a new patient and the patient had a new doctor. We are dynamic. Things change. Reevaluating the patient may be important in making a difficult diagnosis after signs and symptoms have been clarified with the passing of time.

# "YOU'RE REALLY ONE OF THOSE OLD DOCTORS, AREN'T YOU?"

That comment coming from some patients might be considered an insult, but coming from Cathy it was a compliment. Although sixty-seven years old at the time—so chronologically old enough, I prefer to think she meant, "You're really a traditional, old school physician." Her uncle had been a primary care physician in our area and was her model of an "old doctor." Uncle Jack always took time with his patients, knew them personally, and was beloved by them.

Cathy was thirty-two years old, had two children and worked as a nurse on the cardiac care unit (CCU) at the hospital. Like intensive care nurses on other units, she often worked twelve hour shifts. The physically demanding work involved prolonged standing, heavy lifting, and continual use of her hands. A swollen, painful knee was the first sign of rheumatoid arthritis, followed by swelling and morning stiffness in her hands. Mornings are hard on any patient with inflammatory arthritis, but if the morning schedule includes preparing two children for preschool and being at work by 7:00 AM, you have a greater level of difficulty. Fatigue accompanies active inflammation and is exacerbated in the setting of work and family responsibilities.

In rheumatology, we feel there is an urgency in controlling inflammation as soon as possible. Special imaging studies with ultrasound and MRIs have shown erosions beginning early in the course of the disease when routine x-rays may be normal. Control the inflammation and we hope to minimize or avoid the erosive, destructive joint changes of rheumatoid arthritis, as well as decrease pain and improve fatigue (See…"I'm Not Paying For This Visit"). To rapidly control her symptoms, I aspirated and injected her knee with cortisone and started prednisone 5 mg twice a day. She was given information to read on Plaquenil (hydroxychloroquine), the first medicine I would add to hopefully get her illness into remission. This medicine is a weaker DMARD (Disease Modifying Anti-Rheumatic Drug) than meds like methotrexate, but sometimes controls the illness along with vitamin D supplementation and allows a tapering of prednisone. All DMARDs are slow acting agents. Six to twelve weeks might be necessary to see an effect from the Plaquenil. Frequent follow-up is needed to settle on a proper, effective regimen for the individual patient.

I was taught there are three A's of practice. The first and most important is "Availability" followed by "Affability," and finally "Ability." I would add "Affordability" as a fourth "A" in this era of high health care costs. When Cathy returned in two weeks, she was much better and we directed a taper of the prednisone and started Plaquenil. She would need eye check-ups to monitor for possible medication toxicity every six months. We planned to recheck in six weeks, but she called two weeks later. As the prednisone was tapered, her morning stiffness worsened and fluid recurred in her knee. We worked her in on that day's already filled schedule; we were Available.

Some patients are hesitant to call or feel they are imposing on the physician. I always tried to tell the patient I was glad they called and reassured them that I agreed the complaint was important. Affability. Dr. Stead taught that a healthy doctor is never inconvenienced by a sick patient. In Cathy's case, we had to readjust her prednisone taper and re-aspirate and inject her knee. I also asked her to read information we provided for the use of methotrexate, the most common DMARD to start with.

When she returned four weeks later she was better, probably due to the slower taper of prednisone and more time for the Plaquenil and vitamin D supplementation to be effective. I suggested that we add in the methotrexate to achieve a remission. However, the patient and her husband were considering having another child. Methotrexate, as they learned from the handout information, is contraindicated if a couple is trying to conceive or is not on a birth control regimen. With pregnancy concerns, we would give her current regimen more time and consider an alternative DMARD if the RA stayed too active. Ability.

When Cathy was seen eight weeks later in follow-up, she had tapered off prednisone, the RA seemed to be in remission, and she was pregnant. An interesting phenomenon had been noted for years. During pregnancy, RA seems to go into remission or become inactive. An eighty-six-year-old Sunday school classmate, Sharon, had severe RA starting over sixty years ago. Treatment was limited at that time to massive doses of aspirin and real gold shots as the only possible remittive agent. Her husband, E. B., was an accountant at a large company here in Lynchburg. As a number cruncher/bean counter, he calculated they could afford two and three-eighths children. Sharon, however, experienced the only significant relief from her arthritis with the first pregnancy and enjoyed the temporary remission with her second pregnancy, as well. They ended up with five children. Go figure, E. B.

After the third child was born, as expected, Cathy's RA became active again. Now they were ready to get out of the baby business; she had a tubal ligation, and methotrexate was recommended. She, like so many of our patients, had seen ads on TV for the newer biologic agents. Whether golfer Phil Mickelson was plugging Enbrel for psoriatic arthritis or Humira (adalimubab) was being touted for RA, the commercials were similar. Thanks to the litigious nature of our society, patients have to be more scared to death than informed. The first fifteen seconds of the ad tell how great the medicine is—and the next forty-five seconds bring caveats regarding life-threatening infections, cancers, and degenerative brain disease as possible side effects. No placebo effect here.

I explained that in my experience (Ability) we had not seen fatal infections, unusual cancers, nor brain disease in our patients. While we remained concerned and monitored our patients carefully on these meds, the most common side effect was poverty (Affordability). These meds are expensive. Cathy started on the methotrexate and achieved remission. This was maintained on the regimen of generic Plaquenil, folic acid, methotrexate, and vitamin D. My experience over the thirty-five years showed that patients on Plaquenil responded at lower doses of methotrexate with less drug toxicity.

The next time I was referred to as an old doctor was by another rheumatologist—this time at UVa. During my sojourn out of practice from December 31, 2010 to July 2011, I referred a younger female patient, Gina, to UVa for follow-up. At her visit, the patient noted a recurrence of her frequent bronchitis and asked for a prescription of amoxicillin. Once or twice a year, I would need to call in a prescription for her. The attending UVa rheumatologist—who was of the same vintage as me—refused to prescribe an antibiotic, referring Gina to her primary care physician or an urgent care clinic. He explained to the house staff and rheumatology trainees that "some *older* rheumatologists" would do this for their patients, implying that this was not the province nor responsibility of the new, young physician. Doing some primary care for your patients showed more common courtesy than Affability and saved the patient time and money (Affordability). While I'm not glad to be old, I'm proud to be considered "one of those old doctors" by my patients.

# "I KNOW WHAT YOU DOCTORS SAY, BUT…"

Aunt Ruth (the late Mrs. Milton Bush of Salem, West Virginia) could always tell a great story. Humor, energy, and an ability to mimic produced the kind of tales you believed, nodding your head in understanding and agreement. After receiving my medical degree in 1972, the stories were often prefaced with the statement, "Now I know what you doctors say, but…," and a medical anecdote would follow. There was little science supporting her stories but, when this master storyteller finished her tale, you were ready to drink asparagus juice for cancer, stick your hand in the beehive to cure arthritis, or apply Crystal Lake water to your head three times a day and once at night to prevent baldness. Maximum placebo effect was achieved, you heard a good story, and you believed.

I always appreciated the allure of these stories. They were much more convincing and entertaining than medical science. The language was not confused with P values, significance levels, and tables of data. This was practical medical information provided free by a concerned friend, in language you could understand, eminently more believable than the Latin-laden, data loaded, expensive advice given by your doctor in the name of evidence based medicine.

In the late 1970s and early 1980s, my patients were influenced by periodicals like the *Enquirer*. Now TV infomercials and internet searches abound with advice for the arthritis patient. With the already large number of arthritis patients increasing in concert with our aging population, the potential audience presents a lucrative opportunity to sell new meds, topical rubs, copper reinforced joint supports, etc. Sometimes these well-meaning friends and neighbors want you to try a sample of a treatment they are selling as a local agent.

The baby boomers (my wife and I born in 1946 are some of the first boomers) want to preserve their youth, remain active and, as one patient said, "I want to wear out, not rust out." Some of the books touting diets for arthritis and staying young are tremendously popular. Many guarantee results "or your money back."

While there are probably less than 4,000 board certified rheumatologists in our country (compared with ten times more cardiologists), I found that there is no shortage of arthritis experts; one lives beside each of my patients. To doctor and teach my patients most effectively, I acknowledge the lesson from Aunt Ruth. Usually a good story from a friend trumps medical science. I often reached an understanding with my patients. As long as the next "cure for arthritis" was not dangerous or contraindicated with the patient's standard medical regimen, we might give the new med, treatment, rub, diet, or exercise routine a trial over an agreed time period of six to twelve weeks. If no benefit was found, back to our traditional treatment—until the next fad comes out because…"I know what you doctors say, but…"

## "I WANT THAT NEW MEDICINE
## I HEARD ABOUT ON TV"

## (Media and Meds)

Oh, brother. I could see the headlines in the newspaper: "Local Rheumatologist Found Dead on Banks of the Staunton River with Undressed Companion." Thus one of the shortest medical careers in Lynchburg would end in disgrace.

But let me explain. It was May 1980 and striped bass were making the annual spawning run from Buggs Island Lake up the Staunton River. I invited my friend, Dr. J. Russell Rice, to join me for a fishing trip. Russ was one of my main clinical instructors in rheumatology during fellowship training and an avid fisherman and hunter. Driving up from Duke, he would meet me at Brookneal.

The day started well weather-wise but fishless. By midafternoon, however, clouds began gathering and a rumble of thunder announced an approaching storm. Strong wind, heavy rain, and frequent lightning developed quickly and swept down the river. Have you ever been so close to lightning in a thunderstorm that the hair on your arms stood up? When that happened, we knew it was time to head for shore. We planned to settle on the bank and lay low till rain and lightning passed. As I beached the boat, Russ realized he forgot his rain gear and decided to strip down to his underwear, leaving his clothes in a covered compartment on the boat. As we sat there with the thunder and lightning all around us, I imagined the news headlines of a fatal lightning strike.

Fortunately, no catastrophe—but no fish either. Still teaching, Russ asked if I planned to use these new medicines coming out for arthritis. Oraflex (benoxaprofen) and Feldene (piroxicam) were the newest additions to the NSAID (nonsteroidal anti-inflammatory drug) family. I was not inclined to use Oraflex because the product information listed some strange side effects, including a sun-induced redness with peeling of the cuticles, in addition to the usual concerns about gastrointestinal side effects. Feldene's attraction was once-a-day dosing, but it seemed especially likely to cause GI bleeding and the drug had a long half-life. That is, if a problem occurred such as GI bleeding or liver or renal toxicity, the effects of the drug would still be in the patient's system for several days after stopping the med. We agreed these were "me too" drugs rather than significant advances in arthritis treatment. We did not anticipate much use of Oraflex or Feldene. In medicine, you did not want to be the first to embrace the new, nor last to discard the old.

However, that night as Russ headed back to Durham and I drove home to Lynchburg, Walter Cronkite announced on the evening news a major breakthrough in arthritis treatment. Two new medicines—Oraflex and Feldene—were important therapeutic advances. Who could doubt Walter Cronkite? By the time we started practice the next morning, there was no question about using them. Patients called, "I want that new medicine I heard about on TV." You couldn't get samples quickly enough to keep up with the demand. Media trumped our medical judgment. "And that's the way it is," Walter would probably say—and has continued to be.

Our initial hesitancy to embrace the new meds ultimately proved correct. Oraflex was subsequently taken off the market in the U.S. with unacceptable liver toxicity. One of my patients, however, felt that it helped her arthritis more than any other medicine and considered going to Europe for the drug where it was still being prescribed (eventually off the market there, as well).

Feldene has continued to be prescribed and is the number one NSAID related to GI bleeding. This was no surprise as the major risk factor for this complication is age and our population demographics show ever older patients on polypharmacy.

The role of media since the time of my training and early practice has changed greatly. Initially the newspaper or television might announce the arrival of a new med with mild hyperbole. The *Durham Morning Herald* mentioned Clinoril (sulindac) as a medicine that cured spinal arthritis in young men. Not exactly true. It was another NSAID that would be useful in controlling clinical symptoms of ankylosing spondylitis, an inflammatory arthritis often affecting the spinal column in younger male patients, but was not a cure. The main gripe we had as physicians was the medicine being brought to the public's attention before we had been detailed on the new treatment by the drug representative and before we had samples.

Like the Oraflex and Feldene experience, our patients were eager to try the newest medicine, and we saw the zenith of placebo effect. It was wonderful to have samples. As I always told my patients, the purpose of a sample was to allow us to try the medicine and find out, usually over a two-week trial, if the medicine helped and was tolerated. I dreaded my name on the prescription bottle of an expensive new med in my patient's medicine cabinet that wasn't tolerated after the first pill or two. Samples helped avoid this.

Now the emphasis is on direct advertising to the patient. TV, newspapers, magazines, and the Internet are sources encouraging you to "ask your doctor if this new medicine is right for you." From the rheumatology perspective, ads for new biologic arthritis agents follow a similar format. The first part of the commercial tells you how great the medicine is. It controlled their arthritis, allowing them to enjoy almost unrestricted activities: dancing, exercising, recreational sports, and even professional golf. The last part of the commercial delivers the caveats: don't take this medicine if you are allergic to it (how do you know if you've never had it?); fatal infections may occur; there is an increased incidence of cancers and lymphomas, and some patients may experience an unusual brain illness.

The litigious nature of our society requires the disclosure of this information. It's part of the CYP or CYA plan (cover your posterior or cover your assets—if you know what I mean). As a result, the majority of the ad time is spent scaring the patient to death. Articles are now written on the nocebo effect (See…"You and Dr. Burton Were Right"). After reviewing the exhaustive list of all possible side effects, the patient is less likely to tolerate or benefit from the medicine (nocebo).

When providing a sample of a new medicine, I always advised the patient that they could have any side effect under the sun. If they had a new skin rash, mouth sores, flu-like symptoms, stomach upset or anything out of the ordinary after starting the new medicine, stop the medicine and call me. With the advent of too much information priming the nocebo effect, patients often wanted to know which side effect to expect. "None," I would assure them. "Side effects are rare and most likely the new medicine should be well tolerated." Patients are given product information (PI) sheets with their prescriptions listing every conceivable side effect. I often felt that in this nocebo era, I could talk my most severe RA patient out of a potentially very beneficial therapy by emphasizing the litany of possible side effects such that the patient would say, "Thank God I only have this severe arthritis, but at least I won't have one of those terrible side effects." Not the right attitude regarding patient therapy.

Today, the patient's comment would be more like this—"I want that new medicine I heard about on TV—but without any side effects." Believe me, the doctor would like that, too, but it's not likely to happen. There will always be some risk of side effects to weigh against the potential reward of a beneficial therapy. Because, as Walter Cronkite said, "… that's the way it is," and always will be.

# "I DON'T WANT ANY OF THOSE GENETIC DRUGS"

What the patient meant was he didn't want the *generic* substitute for his NSAID (nonsteroidal anti-inflammatory drug). The patient's arthritis was managed well with Voltaren and he was worried that the generic diclofenac might not be as well tolerated or as effective. I reassured him that oversight by the FDA would require that the generic drug met standards of similar tolerance and efficacy as the brand name medication. In most cases, that's so. However, some differences in generic drugs seem to exist.

Over ten years ago, a generic form of Plaquenil (hydroxychloroquine) was developed. This medicine is widely used in rheumatology, especially for patients with rheumatoid arthritis or connective tissue diseases like lupus. It's a derivative of antimalarial medications found over fifty years ago to be helpful for arthritis patients. The main toxicity which concerned physicians was an effect on the eyes. Retinal deposits could affect vision. Until the generics came out, however, there were so few cases of Plaquenil retinal toxicity that the American Ophthalmology Association suggested the patient did not need even a yearly exam to monitor for toxicity. We just did not see this problem.

After brand name Plaquenil came off patent, several pharmaceutical companies manufactured the generic form hydroxychloroquine. All of my patients were switched to the generic form for cost savings. The first concern regarding generic Plaquenil came to my attention when a nurse patient who had been on the medicine for over three years developed an itchy, red rash after starting a generic form made by Mylan. It was unusual to see an allergic skin rash after this long on the medicine. Nevertheless, we stopped the medicine and the rash cleared. Then the nurse proved to be a better investigator than I was. Rather, she did something I didn't have the courage to do. She retried the brand name Plaquenil after the rash had cleared for several weeks. She may have had an extra incentive since her arthritis was becoming more symptomatic off the hydroxychloroquine. She tolerated the brand name Plaquenil without recurrent skin or other allergic reaction and her RA symptoms were improved.

Alerted by this experience, I monitored the clinical course of other patients on generic hydroxychloroquine and decided the Mylan form did not seem as clinically effective and had more toxicity. Other generics seemed okay, but concerns regarding retinal toxicity were more frequent. This might relate to a combination of more sensitive testing, litigious fears, and/or possibly more toxicity of the generic forms. More sensitive automated visual field testing and SD-OCT (spectral density optical coherence tomography—the ophthalmologist always has new gadgets) hopefully pick up retinal toxicity early before severe damage has occurred.

But there is a problem. There is no substitute for hydroxychloroquine. Lupus experts like Dr. John Klippel and Dr. Michelle Petri have felt that the medicine was like an essential daily vitamin for patients with lupus or related connective tissue disorders. As Dr. Petri emphasized so often at our rheumatology meetings—"I hate prednisone, but I love Plaquenil." As her ophthalmology colleagues at Hopkins more frequently were raising the specter of retinal toxicity based on this new sensitive testing, she was wary since, again, there was no equivalent medicine and her extensive experience suggested this was still a rare problem. In my practice, I had been impressed that with optimizing vitamin D therapy I often would decrease the Plaquenil to one a day without clinical worsening. Since toxicity is felt to be related to dosing based on weight (5 mg/kg) and duration of therapy, this may have served as a preventive measure. I had one documented case of Plaquenil eye toxicity in thirty-five years, but an increasing number of recommendations by the ophthalmologist to stop the medicine over the final three years of practice.

More complicated generic meds are on the horizon. The biologic agents for arthritis such as Remicade (infliximab) and Humira (adalimumab) will probably be introduced to the market and will require close monitoring even after FDA approval. Some side effects or adverse reactions won't be apparent until general use. Meanwhile, physicians will need to listen to patients, like my nurse, and remain vigilant in judging efficacy and monitoring for toxicity.

# "I NEED A RIDE"

Our worst fear was realized. Returning from a week in Colorado, Sandra and I found that the last part of our trip, a connecting flight from Dulles to the Lynchburg Airport, was cancelled. It was 10:00 PM. We had started a long exhausting day of travel at 9:00 AM Pacific time. The flight was cancelled because the crew had gone over their allotted hours of flying time. Wouldn't you think that in this time of advanced technology (it was August 9, 2001) the computer might have alerted them so a replacement crew could be arranged? The airline attendant did not seem surprised and certainly showed no remorse.

Sandra and I were especially eager to get home since the next day we would drive to Tuxedo, N.C., to work as counselors at Camp Greystone. An abbreviated five-day week at the end of the summer was an introduction for prospective young campers. Sandra would teach archery and riflery while, as the fishing counselor, I would try to get classes of twelve 8 and 9 year olds through 45 minutes of fishing without hooking each other.

Staying overnight for a flight the next day was not an option. We needed to get home and, in spite of the slowest airport personnel of all time, we got our luggage and fishing rods and headed toward the car rentals. One of our fellow stranded passengers, Barbara S., was not only needing to get home but she appeared to be nine and a half months pregnant. "I need a ride. My husband's at home and commutes to work in Washington. I have to get home to take care of our other two kids." We were glad to offer her a ride, but I warned her that I was a rheumatologist and if she decided to deliver on the way home, we'd both be in trouble. She assured me she wasn't due for another month.

It was after midnight by the time we left. Her husband had arranged for a neighbor to watch the children and the couple shared a mobile phone call as he passed us on the other side of

104

highway 29 headed toward his job at the Pentagon. I counted eleven deer along the roadside coming home, fortunately, not hitting any. It was a relief to get everyone home safely by 3:00 AM.

Sandra and I headed to Camp Greystone in the early afternoon of the next day. Barbara indeed delivered a month later—on September 11, 2001. With Barbara going into labor, her husband stayed home that day instead of making his usual commute to the Pentagon. Imagine the mixed emotions for the family that day: the terror of 9/11 contrasting with the miracle of their child's birth occurring at a time which kept father out of harm's way. What a special celebration for them on 9/11 each year—birthday and thanksgiving.

# "YOU AND DR. BURTON WERE RIGHT"
## (Obecalp/Placebo/Nocebo)

It wasn't easy for Chief Stickley to admit this. He had been opposed to our use of Obecalp (placebo spelled backwards) for those two Navy years (1974-1976). But let me explain.

After a week of orientation to the military at the Norfolk Armed Forces College, our group of physicians received orders for duty stations. "As per BupersMed," I was to "report no later than 0800 1974 July 21 Mayport NavSta comDesron 14." In plain English, I was to report at 8:00 AM on July 21, 1974, to the Mayport Naval Station in Florida, where I would be the GMO (General Medical Officer) for Destroyer Squadron 14. We compared our assignments. Fellow Duke physicians included Bill McClatchey, assigned to an LST out of Norfolk, and Maury Topolosky, who would be in Diego Garcia.

Jay Michael Burton had completed a rotating internship and one year of general surgery residency at the University of Kentucky. He was Kentucky blue through and through, not crazy about Duke, and maintained an accent from his upbringing in West Liberty, Kentucky. Mike was also assigned to Mayport as GMO for DESRON 24. "You're going to have to watch out for Burton. That Kentucky hillbilly doesn't sound too swift," admonished one Duke friend. Mike and I would do the majority of active duty sick call at Mayport over the next year. I would try to keep him out of trouble.

The site of sick call shifted from the Mayport dispensary to large ships such as the *Sanctuary* hospital ship and tenders like the *Grand Canyon*. We were learning Navy medicine. Active duty sick call followed a pattern. There was never a healthy sailor on Monday morning nor a sick one on Friday afternoon. If we had a doubt about a sailor's illness, we would have him come back on Friday. If he was still ailing, we would keep him in the dispensary for observation over the weekend. That threat healed many illnesses.

One Monday morning at the end of sick call on the *Grand Canyon*, Seaman Jones, a corpsman, asked if we could give him something for a persistent headache. He had already tried Tylenol and Darvon Compound. Jones was a solid sailor rising in rank and perhaps heading toward a career in the Navy. He was no hypochondriac nor slacker. Mike and I agreed on a trial of Tylenol #3. Jones returned the next day; no relief. His neurologic exam was normal and we thought it might be a migraine equivalent headache. We would break the cycle with a shot of Demerol. Jones would sleep that day and the headache should be gone by morning. But, no. When he appeared the following day, Mike took over. "You know, there's only one medicine that's going to help. Obecalp." Well, I had trained at a pretty good place, we saw lots of patients with headache problems, we were at the forefront of medical knowledge, and I had never heard of Obecalp.

Mike started his treatment. "Jones, lie down on the stretcher. I'm gonna give you a shot that will put you to sleep for twenty minutes and when you wake up, the headache will be gone and you won't have any drowsy hangover like the Demerol." The needle delivering the 1 cc of sterile saline wasn't even out of his arm and Jones was snoring. He awoke on cue in twenty minutes, headache relieved and no side effects. "You're lucky, Jones. We've got a long acting pill form you can take." We started him on B vitamin pills (chosen because they smelled terrible so must be good medicine) which were kept locked up as a controlled medication, Obecalp, available by prescription only, to be tapered from one every six hours to every twelve hours as needed. This Kentucky Wildcat doctor taught the Dookie a valuable lesson. It's actions, not accents, that count.

In truth, neither Mike nor I made much more of the Obecalp treatment until a month later. Mike was on sea duty and I was finishing sick call. I got an urgent call from Jones. The *Grand Canyon* was going to sea for a Mediterranean cruise. Uh-oh, I thought, this will probably be an attempt to get out of the cruise. The pressure of deployment would reveal that Jones was a psych case and the Obecalp experiment was a fluke. But I was wrong. "Doc Wilson, I need you to write me another prescription for Obecalp. I've tapered it down to one every twelve hours, but if I go longer than that, the headache comes back." He wasn't trying to get out of the cruise, he just wanted to be sure he had his effective medicine. I refilled his prescription and couldn't wait to tell Mike. The Obecalp era had begun.

After he returned from his cruise, Obecalp treatment really took off. We referred to it sometimes as Obecalp Orthopedic, Obecalp Otic, Obecalp Ophthalmic, or Obecalp Pain Reliever depending on the patient's symptoms. It was amazingly effective, and no side effects. As with any medicine, patients would call with suspected adverse reactions. "Doc, since I started the medicine, I've been having some (choose one or more: nausea, vomiting, dizziness, chest pain, shortness of breath, diarrhea, double vision, etc., etc.). Could the Obecalp do this?" Nope. One tenet in our Hippocratic Oath is first do no harm. Obecalp fit the bill and became the number one drug we prescribed.

One day in the midst of sick call, Chief Stickley appeared. "Dr. Wilson and Dr. Burton, I'm here to let you know the dispensary is out of Obecalp." Mike and I looked at each other and burst out laughing. "Chief, how can we be out of nothing?!" Apparently, we had used up the Navy's supply of B vitamins. We switched to little pink placebos and they did as well. The Chief still did not like Obecalp.

The next year the Navy decided to separate Mike and me. That's another story. I had learned by then that Mike was an excellent physician and we became life-long friends. I would spend my second year doing dependent and retired military sick call. Obecalp continued to be a favorite and effective medicine. But one patient bothered me.

A twenty-two year old white female dependent had persistent headaches. Her husband had frequent deployments on an aircraft carrier for extended periods of time. Migraine equivalent or stress related headaches seemed likely. After trying the usual headache medications and some anti-anxiety diazepam, she was given a trial of Obecalp. No better. The patient then decided to see a private doctor in Jacksonville and was lost to follow-up over the next three months.

After seeing several physicians, she was referred to a neurologist and underwent a procedure called a pneumoencephalogram (PEG). This was before the time of CT scans and MRIs. After spinal fluid is drawn off during a lumbar puncture, air is injected and the patient is angled so the air will outline the ventricles of the brain and pick up any irregularities that might suggest brain pathology, like a tumor. One thing for sure, the patient would then experience their worst headache of all time. The patient frequently had to be hospitalized for one or two days to recover, receiving parenteral pain and anti-nausea meds. Her test was normal and the neurologist had run through his gamut of headache meds, all to no avail. Out of frustration, he asked if she *ever* had *any* medicine that helped at all. Guess what? The only medicine that helped even a little was Obecalp. The neurologist looked in his PDR (*Physicians' Desk Reference*) of medications. It was not listed. "I wonder if this is some experimental medicine that only the military has. I'm going to write you a prescription and see if they would be kind enough to fill it for you at the Mayport dispensary."

When the patient showed up with a private physician's prescription for Obecalp, Chief Stickley gave up and came to tell me that Mike and I were right. I couldn't wait to call Mike with the news.

The placebo effect has been defined as improvement in the patient's symptoms that occurs, not because of a particular drug or treatment, but because of the expectations, beliefs, or hopes embedded in the encounter between a patient and a clinician. There has been some debate regarding the use of placebo. Is it honest or ethical? I'll leave that debate for the ethicists. But they sure have been effective. In the past, it was felt that medications and even some procedures had a positive placebo effect at least 30 percent of time.

I have been called a "traditional physician." The patient making the observation implied that I was not sympathetic or attuned to the new age alternative therapies. Certainly, I started out that way. During house-staff training, prior to Navy duty, I was exposed to Dr. Redford Williams. He had completed internal medicine training and was practicing psychiatry and researching psychosomatic studies related to stress. He accompanied us on rounds and, frankly, I thought he was an unnecessary distraction to our delivery of "real medicine." It was with some glee, the second year in the Navy, that I noted an article in the *New England Journal of Medicine* regarding the effect of biofeedback on blood pressure control. A nephrology fellow, Dr. Richard Stone, co-authored the article with Dr. Williams. Like his name, Richard Stone was a rock solid medicine man. No mumbo-jumbo, no psychofluvia. He would prove that all this psychophysiology was bunk. But, no! Without a doubt, the use of biofeedback and stress control helped lower blood pressure more effectively with the same or lesser doses of meds or no meds. Hmmm.

As a rheumatology fellow back at Duke (1978), I was consulting on a pulpwood cutter from eastern North Carolina who was about to lose several fingertips. Perhaps it was Raynaud's phenomenon related to early onset scleroderma or primary Raynaud's aggravated by vibration of his chain saws. The exaggerated vasospasm of the small arteries of the fingers caused impending distal gangrene of several fingertips. Topical nitroglycerin paste to the wrists and directly to fingertips did not help. Intra-arterial reserpine injections likewise were not helpful. One of the house officers asked about biofeedback to control Raynaud's. The cynic in me said, "Are you kidding? First of all, it's black magic, and secondly this fellow's not smart enough to do biofeedback!" Wrong again. Biofeedback worked; it made the vasospasm in the patient's fingertips relax and prevented the loss of fingers. Biofeedback is a way to control the autonomic or automatic nervous system. It has since then proven useful in the management of diverse disorders such as hypertension, irritable bowel syndrome, Raynaud's, fibromyalgia, and general stress related symptoms.

In the early 1970s cardiac catheterization was at least a two-day hospitalization with catheters advanced through cut downs in arms or legs. The studies were carefully reviewed by the entire cardiology team and, if significant coronary artery occlusions were found, the patient was scheduled for a CABG ("cabbage" coronary artery bypass graft). This surgery was in its infancy and, not infrequently, after the patient was anesthetized and had the median sternotomy incision performed, technical equipment problems or intraoperative complications required cancellation of the surgery. Although no bypasses were performed, almost invariably when the patient came out from under anesthesia, angina chest pain symptoms were improved. It was so striking that several times the cardiologists felt the films must have been mislabeled and the patient was studied with a repeat catheterization. The occlusions were still there; over time, symptoms recurred and heart surgery was still needed. But it showed the essence of placebo effect. Even a sham procedure produced impressive temporary symptomatic relief.

What a powerful ally in health care. Whether part of a medication effect (as seen with Obecalp), part of a biofeedback discipline, or temporary effect of surgery, the mind is an important component of health care. The Greeks recognized this since the era of Hippocrates. "Mens sana, corpus sanus." A healthy mind, a healthy body. Dr. Paul Dudley White, a founder and godfather of cardiology, was asked toward the end of his career (1969) if he were starting over again, what field would he pursue? "Psychiatry," was the answer, "because it's at the same stage of infancy as cardiology when I was young and we have so much to learn about the workings of the brain." Still true today.

Skeptics often dismiss responses to complementary and alternative therapies as mere placebo effects in patients who simply misperceived their illness or their recovery. Most doctors, however, believe the placebo effect exists. The mind can make us sick but the placebo effect shows it can be an asset in improving our health. But the beneficial placebo effect is endangered.

Over the last decade there is an increasing nocebo phenomenon in which the patient has expectations of adverse effects at the onset of their treatment. By the time my practice ended (2014), many patients, while being started on a new medicine, wanted to know, "Which side effect(s) should I expect?" "None," I would respond. "Side effects are rare." But this is an increasingly common mindset. There certainly won't be any beneficial placebo effect in these patients.

Where has this come from? A combination of factors have contributed. The more litigious nature of our society and the information age are major causes. Ads for medicines on television and the Internet typically give a brief fifteen second description of the medicine benefits followed by forty-five seconds off fear.

Ads for the biologic arthritis therapies are a good example. After telling how beneficial a medicine like Humira might be for a patient with severe rheumatoid arthritis (RA), the caveats begin. "Don't take Humira if you're allergic to it." How do you know if you've never taken the medicine? "This medicine may increase your susceptibility to serious and possibly fatal infections. Let your doctor know if you are from an area of fungal infections." How many patients are aware of fungal diseases like histoplasmosis or blastomycosis in their region? "There may be an increased incidence of cancer, especially lymphomas in patients taking this medicine." Actually, patients with RA have a higher frequency of lymphomas unrelated to any medicine. "Some patients may develop a brain disorder called PML (Progressive Multifocal Leukoencephalopathy), which is usually fatal.

So, let's see. Your arthritis may be improved if you don't die of infection, cancer, or brain disease. In over a decade of using these agents I have never had a patient with any of these fatal outcomes. But I had many patients decline a biologic agent. Their attitude was, "Thank heaven all I have is this painful disabling arthritis. At least I won't have any of those terrible side effects." But we missed the opportunity for a potentially beneficial treatment.

Why do the drug companies feel they have to publicize these rare adverse drug reactions? Thank our lawyers. The companies are using a CYA strategy—Cover Your Ass(ets.) The class action suits are too great a threat. We saw this years ago when many of the drug companies were not going to manufacture vaccines due to liability concerns. Between the lawyers and the media, none of us will die a natural death. We'll be scared to death and die of anxiety and fear. We are ripe for the nocebo effect as placebo benefits gradually diminish.

I miss Obecalp.

# "WHEN YOU TAKE CARE OF MOM
# YOU TAKE CARE OF THE WHOLE FAMILY"

## (Fibromyalgia)

Jan's comment made me think of the T-shirt message—"If momma ain't happy, nobody's happy." Probably deservedly so. I had followed Jan in the office for twenty-two years, beginning when she was an eighteen-year-old college student. She had a history of juvenile rheumatoid arthritis with some residual activity of arthritis into adulthood. Over the years, I had the opportunity to see her as a college student, young single working at her first job as a receptionist at a dentist's office, newlywed, young mother, and now a mature forty-year-old mother of two boys, balancing duties of mother, wife, and paralegal. Her plate was full. The boys were approaching teenage—God's final exam of parenting, and there was plenty of stress. Sometimes aches and pains corresponded to arthritis flare-ups, at other times acting like a stress-related fibromyalgia flare or a combination of the two.

Jan demonstrated the perfect set of factors for fibromyalgia. Stresses at work, motherhood, housewife duties, and inflammatory arthritis can be overwhelming. Picture fibromyalgia as a cycle. Musculoskeletal pains (arthralgia and myalgias) interrupt the restorative non-REM (rapid eye movement) phase of sleep, resulting in a decrease in the body's natural painkillers (endorphins). Decreased endorphins result in more pain and the cycle repeats.

Can the cycle be broken with arthritis meds like ibuprofen or naproxen? Rarely. Sometimes, low doses of meds like amitriptyline will help the sleep cycle. Aerobic exercise can increase endorphins (part of the explanation of the jogger's high), but it's hard to exercise when you already hurt all over, and Mom often has no time in an already busy schedule.

I also consider fibromyalgia a disease of our time. It's almost impossible to go through a twenty-four-hour period without being aware of all the miseries in our world. Availability of news 24/7 feeds a compulsion to be informed, yet the information fed into our personal computer brain produces an exercise in frustration and futility; we are powerless to do anything about it other than worry and ache.

So, why is this worse in women? Society places different expectations on men and women. A man's orientation of responsibilities is vertically oriented. I picture a protective umbrella over a list of job, family, and home responsibilities. If a man lets his grass grow too high, or trash gets out of hand, house gets into a state of disrepair, or he misses dinner or his kid's Little League games, society is forgiving. Old Joe is working so hard; he's had a lot of pressure at work; it's okay for him to let these other things go. First priority is his work and that is his protective umbrella.

The mom's responsibilities are horizontally oriented. No single duty acts as a protective umbrella or excuse. Picture the old Ed Sullivan shows when a performer balanced spinning plates on sticks. He continued to add additional plates and stick set-ups while running up and down to keep the plates moving and balanced. This is mom's dilemma. Society puts equal weight on career, mother, homemaker duties. It's not okay to let the house get filthy, forget the kids' dental appointments, be late for work, skip school activities, get fast food for dinner every night, and be too tired for marital relations. Not fair, but true. No protective umbrella for mom.

Fibromyalgia is a spectrum of diseases. In its mildest form, a temporary worry like your upcoming IRS audit interrupts your sleep and you awake with body aches, which leave when the audit is over. More typical would be conditions like Jan's. Control of inflammation and modification of sleep with low dose amitriptyline may free the patient up for aerobic exercise as endorphins build up.

At the far end of the spectrum, however, are psychological problems manifested by fibromyalgia aches and pains. One academic rheumatology professor, Dr. John Winfield, found that 30 percent of these patients had a history of childhood abuse—physical, sexual, or mental. These patients may benefit with professional psychiatric or psychological counseling.

Fortunately, in Jan's case, controlling her inflammatory arthritis and taking a low dose of amitriptyline at night brought things back in line. Kids, husband, neighbors, and friends at work were all happier. Jan was right. When you take care of mom, you take care of the whole family.

# "YOU'RE THE DOC"

What a gratifying comment. Eugene Morris and I had been fighting his arthritis for over thirty years. During that time, we tried all the standard therapies: NSAIDs (Nonsteroidal Anti-Inflammatory Drugs) including Butazolidine (phenylbutazone), which was taken off the market, steroids, DMARDs (Disease Modifying Anti-Rheumatic Drugs such as gold shots, methotrexate, azathioprine, cyclophosphamide). All failed. New biologic agents had come on the market and I was recommending etanercept (Enbrel). After going over the usual warnings of fatal infection, induced cancers, and a fatal brain illness, I wouldn't blame Eugene if he decided to pass. But he was going to try this new medicine simply because I suggested it…"You're the doc."

If a doctor wants honest and insightful feedback on his patient/physician relationship, I found the best way to do this. Forget a questionnaire or post-visit email evaluation; put your mother in the waiting room as a fellow patient. My mother was in the office for a knee injection, sharing the wait with Eugene. A new patient had an appointment and asked Eugene how long he'd been seeing me and if I had helped him. "For over twenty years" and "No, but he keeps on trying." Mom couldn't wait to share that story with me. And it was true. Hadn't helped him as much as we hoped, but we kept on trying.

The attitude "You're the doc, we'll do whatever you suggest" is something a physician does not take lightly. The patient is giving the doctor *authority* in his care decisions. It not only represents a recognition of the doctor's knowledge but, more importantly, a trust that the doctor will weigh all factors in deciding what is best for the patient. With that authority comes the *responsibility* to serve as the patient's advocate and fiduciary. Eugene and the majority of my central Virginia patients were like this. As a physician, I feel an *ownership* of this patient's medical problem; no one knows the patient better nor cares more about him. Failure of one treatment is not a reason for accepting defeat and giving up. When you feel an ownership of the patient, you keep on trying.

*Ownership* I liken to the concept of *dominion* in Genesis 1:26. "...let them have dominion over the fish of the sea, and over the birds of the air, and over the cattle, and over all the earth..." Dominion is not ruling with unquestioned authority for your own benefit but, rather, is the ultimate responsibility calling for you to be a good steward, recognizing and caring for a special resource—your patient.

Unfortunately, there is an increasing disconnect between authority and responsibility. The physician's authority is challenged and eroded on all sides. The health insurers question tests and treatments. An MRI of the back may not be paid for until the patient has completed a course of physical therapy; a new biologic won't be covered unless the patient has failed on methotrexate and a different biologic. Challenging the health insurance company takes time, interrupts the clinical schedule, and often requires calls directly from the physician for peer review. Yet, if there is delay or failure to diagnose cancer because an MRI was not approved or the patient has a fatal reaction to a biologic the health insurer required, who do you think is held responsible?

Physicians employed by hospital systems have economic credentialing reviews. If the patient's length of stay is too long, it may cost the hospital system money. In DRG (Diagnosis Related Group) compensation, the physician was pressured to discharge the Medicare patient as soon as possible. If the patient had pneumonia, they may have coverage for five days. If the patient went home in three days, the hospital made money. Patients were sent home sooner and sicker. If there was a problem, simply readmit them. Now Medicare has caught on to the "home sooner and sicker" readmit strategy with the result of a more dangerous incentive to deny illness or failed treatment when the patient shows up too soon in the ER after discharge. One gambit now is to hold the patient up to three days in an outpatient status to avoid readmission which is monitored by Medicare.

An example of the authority-responsibility disconnect affecting one of my fellow physicians involved an eighty-five-year old man with urosepsis—infection from the urinary tract into the blood stream. Each day the hospital reviewers encouraged the physician to discharge the patient. On the day of discharge, cloudy urine was seen in his catheter and bag. The patient's granddaughter worked as a nurse at the hospital. In spite of cloudy urine, suggesting active infection, the patient was discharged to a nursing facility, only to be admitted two days later with overwhelming and fatal infection. While the doctor's authority in keeping the patient hospitalized was challenged each day by the Medicare hospital reviewers, the hospital's final argument was to deny any fault since only a doctor can discharge a patient. It was the doctor's responsibility. With this prevailing authority-responsibility disconnect, it is no wonder the physician does not feel ownership of the patient.

Even more reason to relish Eugene's response. The Enbrel worked beautifully. I wish we had it available twenty years earlier. How nice it would be to answer queries from insurance companies, Medicare, or the hospital regarding patient-related testing, treatment, or length of stay with a terse: "Because I said so."

And their response like Eugene's, "OK, you're the doc."

# "I DON'T LIKE THAT NEW ELECTRIC RECORD"
## (Electronic Medical Record—EMR)

What Bill meant was he didn't like the new electronic health record (EHR) or electronic medical record (EMR). Last week he had an office visit with his primary physician to follow his high blood pressure and elevated cholesterol. The doctor was so focused on documenting information in the EMR that he never looked directly at Bill. After a cursory physical examination, Bill mentioned that he was having some stomach pains. Sorry. He would have to make a separate appointment to address this new problem: he was there just for evaluation of high blood pressure and hyperlipidemia.

The lack of personal interaction between physician and patient is a common complaint since the EMR has become more widely used. A TV commercial by Athena Health parodies the problem. A husband and wife look in on their young son who is typing on his laptop. "Oh, look," the proud mother gushes, "he's playing doctor." As the parents start to interject a comment to the child, their son looks up and raises a finger to hush them as he turns back to the computer.

The EMR is reminiscent of HIPAA. Initial goals are good, but not realized. Few patients or doctors remember what the "HIP" of HIPAA stands for: Health Insurance Portability. In this time when young people may change jobs frequently, the benefit of health insurance portability is obvious. Pre-existing conditions in the individual or a dependent should not hinder their chance to pursue new work opportunities. This was in force before Obamacare, but was touted again as a benefit of the Affordable Care Act (ACA) with the promise the individual could keep the plan he or she liked albeit at higher premium rates, deductibles, and co-pays. HIPAA has mainly become a privacy issue and a periodic nuisance frequently updated at each doctor's office.

The EMR ideally would have all patient medical information readily available on a shared record with all lab and special study results documented. It would keep us from repeating tests already checked. In reality, the EMR systems often do not interact between physician offices or hospitals and offices. The individual record has mistaken quantity of information for quality. Searching through the mass of information is inefficient. As a subspecialist, patients were often referred to me with forty or more pages of faxed EMR notes. This was easier for the referring physician than dictating a thoughtful referral note outlining the patient's problem and relevant test results. I remember one patient coming in with sixty-six pages of copied EMR and wondering why I couldn't review them at the time of the visit or later after office hours. I asked her to take sixty-six pages of information to her lawyer and see if he would review it in a fifteen-minute visit or at home for free.

I worked with two EMR systems. Penchart by Amicore was the first system at Lynchburg Rheumatology Clinic and Allscripts was used my last three years of practice with Rheumatology of CVFP. I refused to carry a laptop into the room when seeing my patients. I wanted to see the expression on their faces as we discussed their problems. I would take notes on my clipboard and run back to the office to document for the EMR. I did not have a scribe and still feel that the most important training I received for using the EMR was in summer school 1961 when my mother made me take a typing class. I became my own transcriptionist.

If I wanted to save health care expenditures in the guise of improving quality, I would propose the EMR. It makes the physician less efficient—one study found that the EMR added four hours of uncompensated work to the physician's week. I suspect more. Many of my fellow physicians were routinely spending hours each night finishing EMR notes after the office closed.

Progressive government requirements also hobble the operation. Electronic prescribing ("E" prescribing) was an early requirement. This would have required an upgrade of my first

EMR costing $30,000. In more recent times, "meaningful use" (read "meaningless") has gone from reasonable standards such as asking about smoking and following up on elevated BP to ridiculous measures. In my final year of practice, I was told I had met the meaningful use criteria for childhood asthma. Nice, but surprising, since I had not seen any patients with childhood asthma. I suppose I also met meaningful use criteria for brain surgery.

One euphemism regarding the EMR is the claim to be a paperless record. Yet, each patient was sent out with several sheets of paper summarizing problems, ordered tests, and prescriptions. Faxed records included sheets and sheets of worthless information in place of a thoughtful referral note. Finding relevant material in the mass of paper is like the game Finding Waldo. In the name of paperless, there won't be one tree left standing.

The EMR provides a disincentive for investigating problems. As Bill found, the doctor did not want to hear about any problems beyond the BP and cholesterol. More problems would require further documentation and time. So another problem? Another appointment. If the patient is worried and wants more immediate attention, he may be directed to an urgent care center or the ER where he will likely be seen by a physician who does not know the patient and most likely the facility will not have access to a shared EMR.

There is also the concept of dismissal. "I don't know what you have, but it's not in my field." The increasingly impersonal nature of the EMR has destroyed the doctor's sense of ownership of the patient and his problems. This is aggravated by the disconnect of authority and responsibility (See..."You're The Doc"). The doctor's authority is increasingly challenged by insurance companies, hospital systems, and the government. Yet the physician is left with the responsibility for the patient. No wonder the doctor doesn't want to pursue or investigate other complaints.

Bill's disenchantment with the EMR translated to dissatisfaction with his doctor. He's trying to find a new physician who will treat him rather than the laptop. Good luck.

# "I DON'T WANT TO END UP LIKE THAT"

Paul had missed the point. His remark came after our rheumatoid arthritis (RA) support group meeting. Everyone had left and he was referring to Susan, a seventy-four-year-old with long-standing, severely deforming arthritis. The intent or point of the meeting was to have patients with similar illnesses exchange ideas for coping with a chronic illness, like RA. His fearful reaction assured compliance with his medical treatment, but he would not benefit with an insight into the spirit of patients like Susan.

I felt a special connection. Any patient sharing my West Virginia roots was referred to as "cousin." We had lived with the "first cousin" jokes. Do you know why there's no DNA evidence in West Virginia crime investigations? Because all the DNA's the same. Inbreeding. Do you know why it's good the toothbrush was invented in West Virginia? Because, otherwise, it would be called the _teeth_brush. What's the similarity of a West Virginia divorce and a tornado in Oklahoma? In both cases someone loses a double-wide trailer.

Okay, enough. But beyond both of us bearing the brunt of these jokes, Susan was special because she came from Charleston, West Virginia, widow of a prominent judge and lived there about the time my brother and I were born. Susan and her husband were contemporaries of my parents. Their paths had crossed briefly with activities like bridge club socials before my family moved on.

Susan lived the next forty years in Charleston. She and the judge did not have any children; her only relative was a brother and his family in Colorado. Susan's RA progressed in spite of standard treatments used in the 1950s and 1960s. She was severely disabled at the time her husband died. She coped for two years after his death with the help of friends before moving to Lynchburg.

Physical disability was not accompanied by mental or spiritual disability. Just like my mother, Susan's West Virginia roots included a strong desire to be independent as long as possible and not be a burden on family or friends. She came to Westminster Canterbury (WC) a CCRC (continuous care retirement community) soon after it opened. Pride, determination, spirit and the eventual 24/7 care by a wonderful aide, Edith, allowed her to continue independent living in her small apartment.

After an article appeared in the *News & Advance,* Sandra and I decided to expand our West Virginia family connections. The newspaper story related how Susan did not feel welcomed with open arms and compassion. She was embarrassed by her physical disabilities and sensed that some fellow residents felt uncomfortable around her. Perhaps they had a fear like Paul's— would I end up like that? None of us like to be reminded of, or given preview of, eventual physical frailties and disabilities.

With her family so far away and travel becoming more difficult physically, we began to include Susan at family get-togethers, especially at holiday time. Thanksgiving and Christmas dinners were a special celebration with the addition of "Cousin" Susan. I would usually pick her up at WC and deliver her back home that evening. She was a gift for us enjoyed by Sandra, our preteen daughters, Elizabeth and Melissa, and me. She often sent flowers as a table centerpiece, and enlivened conversation with West Virginia stories. She enjoyed the family, including Muffet, our miniature poodle, who reminded her of a beloved Airedale terrier. We even arranged a meal together when my mother was visiting from Parkersburg so they could recall Charleston days.

Outside of office visits, occasional hospitalizations (one case of facial and ocular shingles), and dinners, Susan became more and more apartment bound. One of her pleasures, reading, was threatened with advancing macular degeneration. This was about the time books on tape and recorded newspaper readings became available. Sandra, with her library science background, helped organize tapes and a machine for listening. Disabilities progressed, including an amputation of one leg due to peripheral artery disease. When transportation for office visits became too difficult and exhausting, I began making house or, rather, apartment calls.

Over these six years of personal and professional interaction with Susan, I never witnessed any self-pity. She was what I call "West Virginia" and "rheumatology" strong (before we knew about "Boston" strong). Pride, resilience, independence, courage—all qualities I would witness for years in many patients—were never more magnificently manifested than by Susan.

House calls, office visits, hospitalizations, and holiday get-togethers were a joy, never a burden. I was privileged to care for her in life and even at the time of her death. A call came to the office just as morning appointments were ending. Susan had arrested in the WC beauty parlor, CPR had been started, and she was being transported to Lynchburg General ER. When I arrived at the ER, she had been intubated and chest compressions were under way. EKG showed asystole—no spontaneous heartbeats. Pupils were fixed and dilated. We could try intracardiac epinephrine injection; put in a pacemaker; perhaps stabilize her on a respirator in the ICU. But Susan was giving me one more lesson—the difference in what we could do and should do. Stop the CPR.

I asked to be alone with Susan after tubes and IVs were removed. Tearing up a little, I said goodbye and reflected on the journey we shared and what Susan represented to me: patient, friend, honorary cousin, and mentor, showing us the humanity and spirit wrapped in a deformed and disabled body. While Paul was correct in some regards—we don't want to end up in the physical condition Susan experienced, we need to witness and remember her spiritual state and strong character. We should hope to end up that way—West Virginia strong.

# "HE'S GONE"
## (Dermatomyositis and the Old School Nurse)

I sprang out of the stairwell onto Krise 5 and headed toward John's room. Marie Evans, the floor charge nurse, was waiting for me. As we ran down the hall, she hit me with the news, "It's too late, he's gone."

Fifteen minutes earlier, I had been awakened at home by the answering service. "Call Krise 5 as soon as possible." Mrs. Evans answered the phone. "I'm sorry to call so late (around 2:00 AM), but I'm worried about Mr. Davidson. He just doesn't look good."

Enough said. Mrs. Evans was an old school nurse with over forty years of patient care experience. I did not need a run down on current vital signs or recent lab tests. If she called, worried about a patient, you jumped out of bed, pulled on your clothes and got to the hospital. Her concerns were always justified.

This time, fortunately, she was wrong. While John Davidson (J. D.) was seriously ill as she suspected, he was not gone—although *nearly* gone. Opening the crash cart, I started the ABC's of CPR. Airway first. As I extended his neck back, advanced the laryngoscope, and began intubation, J. D. sputtered and coughed. The procedure must have stimulated a reflex reaction. For whatever reason, his heart rhythm returned with atrial fibrillation and he began breathing spontaneously. We stabilized the patient and transferred J. D. to the MICU (Medical Intensive Care Unit).

J. D. had a complicated case of dermatomyositis. This autoimmune member of the connective tissue disorders (cousin of lupus) involved inflammatory muscle disease with weakness in muscles, skin rash, sometimes associated occult cancers, and often lung problems. If the patient doesn't respond to high dose steroids, the physician adds immunosuppressive meds like

127

azathioprine (Imuran). J. D. had not responded and I sent him to Duke for medical center input. On their recommendation, when he returned to Virginia Baptist Hospital (VBH), we decided to try intravenous cyclophosphamide along with steroids. The dermatomyositis had affected his swallowing muscles. He was losing weight, in a state of inanition, and prone to aspiration.

As lab studies came back after John's admission to the MICU, the events leading up to his arrest were becoming clear. Blood studies showed severe anemia with a hemoglobin of 2 gm/dl (should be 13) and hematocrit of 6 (normal 40). Nasogastric (NG) tube drainage showed fresh blood. J. D. had a stress ulcer causing a GI bleed resulting in hematemesis (vomiting blood) and aspiration leading to the arrest. IV fluids and six blood transfusions over the next two days stabilized his condition. Cyclophosphamide was stopped. Then something strange occurred.

Dermatomyositis caused increased CK (creatine kinase) levels. The higher levels usually correlate with muscle weakness and disease activity. His level had remained around 3000 IU/L (normal 45-180 IU/L) unaffected by the steroids, azathioprine or cyclophosphamide. But over the next six weeks, the CK level came down to normal levels and his muscle strength returned. My consulting rheumatologists at Duke were likewise amazed. I wonder if, in effect, we exchange transfused him. The GI bleed may have been a mixed blessing. Since this time (1981), plasmaphoresis has been used in various autoimmune conditions removing harmful immunoglobulins. Maybe J. D.'s multiple transfusions did something similar.

For whatever reason, over the next year as he followed up in the office, there was no evidence of active dermatomyositis and all medications were stopped. Although his course in the hospital and especially in the MICU had been difficult, he remembered almost none of it—the blessing of retrograde amnesia. But he did remember his nurses, most especially Mrs. Evans.

During my thirty-five years of practice in Lynchburg, my patients and I were blessed with magnificent nurses. I fondly remember several nurses of the same vintage as Mrs. Evans who were likewise dedicated to caring for and caring about patients. Nurses Gilchrist, Bowman, and Harris come to mind.

I differentiate "caring for" (providing medical or nursing services) from "caring about"—an intangible quality combining professional commitment and personal concern that may not be measurable, quantitated, or qualified. It reminds me of the comment attributed to Supreme Court Justice Hugo Black regarding pornography. "I can't define it, but I know it when I see it." And the patients knew this special caring when they received it. These nurses were in touch with their patients. If one of them expressed a particular concern about your patient, you knew it deserved special attention. They looked forward to rounding with the attending physician. It was a chance to learn and clarify any questions regarding that patient's scheduled tests or treatments.

Several of the "Old School" nurses became my patients over the years. At office visits they often expressed frustration as they found themselves spending more time with a computer than with their patients. Instead of accompanying the attending physician on rounds with patient charts, the nurse was what I called "dancing with McKesson"—walking the halls holding onto the McKesson nursing computer cart. Priority was given to documenting all their activities. They were realizing the caveat that not all important things can be documented, and not all things documented are important (See..."I Don't Like That Electric Record").

The ultimate example of computer care trumping patient care was demonstrated one Wednesday morning on rounds. A fellow physician was talking with his partner, expressing chagrin and some anger. He had been called at the office by a patient's family. "Why haven't you seen Mom in the hospital?" Because he didn't know she was there.

His patient was admitted late Sunday night on the preceding weekend. The on-call physician was notified and holding orders were written by the ER physician, a courtesy for the physician taking calls for their practice that weekend. However, Mom's physician was never told about the admission. For the next three days, the ER doctor's orders were followed, the nurses documented everything correctly, and the only thing missing was a doctor. The patient and her family had a healthy chart, but they still wanted her doctor in the picture.

Maybe Mrs. Evans's comment now relates to the personal physician in this time of EMRs, documentation, and health care providers, such as hospitalists, physician assistants and nurse practitioners—"He's gone!"

# "YOU MUST HAVE DONE SOMETHING RIGHT"

## (Statin Myopathy—Treating Gout)

I had followed L. G., a seventy-two-year-old black male for the last five years. He was commenting on something that delighted both of us. Hand and elbow deformities from long-standing gout were shrinking away and the muscle strength in his legs was improving.

He had a complicated history. Thirty-five years of gout treated only episodically for flares had left tophaceous deposits of urate in fingers and elbows causing RA (rheumatoid arthritis)-like deformities with pain and impaired use of hands and arms. He had taken allopurinol for only a short time in the past. He should have been on it chronically.

L. G. demonstrated two things about gout: (1) it can be as disabling and deforming as RA, and (2) the treatment of acute flares is different than intercritical (between flares) and chronic treatment. With an acute attack of gout, a combination of medicines such as colchicine, oral and injectable steroids, and pain meds may be needed. But one thing you don't use acutely is allopurinol. That will mobilize the uric acid in the body and worsen acute gout. After controlling the acute episode, you slowly taper down the steroids and continue long term colchicine (usually 0.6 mg two times daily). When the acute inflammation is controlled, allopurinol is introduced slowly starting at 50 mg daily increasing over six or eight weeks to 300 mg daily (intercritical treatment phase). At this time, taper completely off the prednisone and colchicine, using allopurinol alone (aiming for serum uric acid level <6 mg/dl). Keep colchicine on hand for use as needed if a twinge of acute gout is felt (for instance following your July 4th weenie roast and beer fest).

L. G. had chronic kidney trouble resulting from the most severe reaction possible with statin medications. The meds are lifesavers by controlling cholesterol levels and decreasing heart attacks, but many patients have myalgias (muscle aches) when taking these meds, often associated with a slight elevation of serum CK (creatine kinase) level indicating drug-induced inflammation of the muscles. Rarely, a patient like L. G. may have diffuse breakdown of muscle, called rhabdomyolysis, which can cause severe weakness and kidney failure. This had occurred and after months of treatment, including temporary dialysis, he was left with renal insufficiency and residual weakness in proximal leg muscles which impaired walking and rising from a seated position. He still had active muscle inflammation with CK of 600 mg/dl (normal <180 mg/dl) and what I call smoldering gout—still painful at times with persistent deformities. He needed prednisone for active inflammation in muscles and joints, as well as colchicine for active gout and to prevent flares as we began chronic therapy. Due to residual renal insufficiency, we cautiously introduced febuxostat (Uloric) 20 mg daily. Colchicine may rarely cause myopathy as a side effect so this was watched carefully as we tapered down his prednisone.

Over the next few years, the gouty swellings decreased in size, hand pain lessened, manual dexterity improved, and there was less leg weakness. The Uloric was tolerated and allowed colchicine use only as needed and prednisone was stopped. At his last visit, L. G. and I celebrated as we reviewed x-ray changes in the hands showing filled in gouty defects of the bones and disappearing tophi.

Indeed, I "must have done something right." His comment reminded me of my wife's news one evening. "I ran into one of your patients today. She said you actually helped her." Sandra sounded surprised. As I reminded L. G.—don't be so surprised.

Probably of more importance to L. G. was the relationship of pharmacogenetics to statin sensitivity and vitamin D metabolism. There is an inherited tendency for diseases (See… "Your Father Took Care of My Mother") and for drug metabolism and toxicity. A study in the *New England Journal of Medicine*,

August 21, 2008, showed the association of a genetic variant (SLCO1B1) with statin-induced myopathy. A follow-up article in the *Journal of the American Medical Association,* January 21, 2009, found that variant responsible for 60 percent of 85 myopathy cases they studied. An article in the *Lancet,* July 17, 2010, discussed common genetic determinants of Vitamin D insufficiency. This explained my observation over the last fifteen years of family members with low Vitamin D levels and similar response to replacement regimens.

As with L. G., I encourage my patients to serve as their family champion. Inform all the relatives about these inherited tendencies. If we prevent severe reactions to statins and guide Vitamin D therapy in other family members, then we really must have done something right together.

# "I HOPE I DIE BEFORE YOU RETIRE"

Be careful what you ask for. Frances Lawhorne was eighty-six years old when she expressed this wish. She had over forty years of severe deforming RA (rheumatoid arthritis) and by the time I first saw her in 1983, the disease had ravaged her body. Multiple joint replacements and osteoporosis made each step an adventure and getting upright from a sitting or reclining position was a two or three person exercise. Built-up handles on spoons and forks were necessary for even rudimentary hand grip. In short, she had long-standing problems with little to offer from current therapies. Unfortunately, by the time we saw some of these patients, the cow was already out of the barn. Opportunities had been lost.

So why did she want her demise to precede my retirement? She summed it up well. "I just always feel better when I see you." Injections of steroids—intraarticular and systemic, seemed to help briefly, but I think she felt special with the attention she obtained from our entire staff. We admired her spirit (See..."I Don't Want to End Up Like That"). In spite of her own infirmity, she took care of her husband through his terminal illness from myeloma. Not an easy chore.

Our entire staff went to her ninetieth birthday party held at Fairview United Methodist Church, the church she and her husband attended and supported for years. We presented a mock injection syringe as a gag gift. I had seen other family members with inherited familial arthritis problems and felt like a family doctor. One time when she had a possible skin infection, I asked, "Who's your primary doctor?" "Why you, of course," she answered. I was simultaneously promoted and honored.

Over the next few years, she became more housebound and feeble. Linda Lawhorne, her daughter here in Lynchburg, was the primary caregiver. Trips to the office were too difficult and I made an occasional house call for an injection. It's always interesting to visit a patient's home. It provides a whole new dimension in the doctor-patient relationship. Unfortunately, I'm afraid the house call is on the endangered list if not extinct. Too bad.

On one of these visits, she repeated her wish. I told her she'd have to live at least to one hundred since I had no plans to retire soon. Frances didn't make it, nor did I. Spinal stenosis surgery in late 2012 slowed me down and the onset of Parkinson's brought on retirement in December 2014. Now the doctor, as a patient, has taken his cue from Frances. I don't want my primary physician or neurologist to retire before I die. Not so much a macabre wish but another valuable and practical lesson a special patient taught me.

# "YOU'VE GOT A WORK-IN"

The schedule was full that October morning. Just as I emerged from exam room #1, having seen what I assumed was my last patient for the morning, I spied a record in the chart rack of exam room 2—"Work-in; possible gout." I had a mixed reaction. Disappointed, thinking morning clinic was finished, but accepting since acute gout can be a true emergency, and my office staff usually decided correctly when a patient needed to be seen as an urgent work-in.

I opened the door. The patient was lying on the table, sheet over her body and a hideous, giant, green rubber foot dangling over the edge of the table. I should have known. It was almost Halloween and Jenny was making her annual visit dressed up in full monster regalia. Her daughter came along dressed as a sister witch. Halloween tricks and treats were exchanged and I threatened to inject her artificial foot. For years, residing on my credenza was a large syringe filled with Sweet Tarts, a Christmas gift crafted by Jenny in honor of my fondness for injecting joints. We had a great relationship trading saucy remarks during her visits. Whenever I got ready to inject I'd say, "Now you're going to get it!" Her retort? "You better not hurt me!"

Work-ins are usually not as entertaining as Jenny. In teaching Family Practice residents and medical students, I tried to get them psyched up for the work-in patient. "It's someone with an acute problem, which you can help with." "They may need an x-ray or injection." "Yes, they always seem to come at an inopportune time." "Try to think in economic terms. Pretend this patient is presenting right after you've paid your overhead for the day—pure profit."

Dr. Eugene Stead, Jr., a godfather of internal medicine training, always taught us that a healthy doctor is not inconvenienced by a sick patient. It's more difficult to maintain this perspective in the era of the EMR (Electronic Medical Record) when extensive documentation is required. A simple work-in for bursitis used to be a short note: "Pt woke with pain in R shoulder. Similar episode in past. No hx of injury. Pain on abduction. X-ray shows calcific deposit. Probable calcific tendinitis. Injected and patient instructed in exercises. Return as needed." The EMR would expand the note at least three-fold listing a myriad of things that were not present nor relevant. If the work-in had a complicated problem like a flare of lupus or vasculitis, the documentation could be extensive and time consuming. The result? It's much more difficult to be worked-in at the doctor's office. Instead, the patient is frequently shunted off to the ER or an urgent care center missing continuity of care with the physician who knows him or her best.

I was gratified in the spring of 2005 when a medical student, Kate Mitchell, spent two weeks at the office. Kate is the daughter of John and Dale Lawrence. John and I were in med school and house staff training together. He was a founding physician of the large cardiology practice in Asheville. He wanted his daughter to see a working clinical rheumatology practice. John felt that she probably could not manage a rigorous cardiology practice, but could handle the simple, less demanding rheumatology life. Okay, I accepted that mild slur and still looked forward to introducing her to my rheumatology clinic.

I was "gratified" because Kate just "got it." Maybe her experience as a patient her freshman year at Duke with a serious case of Hodgkins helped her relate to patients with compassion and understanding that I have rarely seen in young doctors. She summarized her experience in a thoughtful note which included the following: "As a student, I love collecting 'Pearls'. During the short time that I was with you I learned (among other things): (1) Learn to juggle two rooms—it increases your efficiency; (2) Show your patients their films—it helps them understand their condition; (3) Talk to your new patients in your personal office (I had never seen this done before. I thought it brought "dignity to the occasion"); (4) Work-ins are *Fun*! Be Flexible!"

Kate completed her post-graduate medical training (internship and residency in internal medicine) at Duke followed by a rheumatology fellowship. I've often thought that my greatest contribution to rheumatology was influencing her in that direction—and, of course, saving her from a demanding cardiology career. I hope her work-ins and practice always remain fun.

Addendum: Jenny was killed in an automobile accident when an on-coming car crossed into her lane. Patients like her enriched my practice, are missed, and remain fondly remembered.

# "DON'T TEACH ME SOMETHING THAT WON'T BE TRUE TWO YEARS FROM NOW"

Maybe the way the comment was addressed intimidated me as much as the doctor who delivered it. "**Mister** Wilson, don't teach me something that won't be true two years from now." It was the first of many things I would learn from Dr. Eugene A. Stead, Jr. over the years. Did the title "Mister" suggest that I might not become **Dr.** Wilson? Let me explain.

As a second year medical student, I tried to avoid Dr. Stead. Stories of second and even fourth-year students being brought to tears during patient presentations to the past Chairman of the Department of Medicine, frankly, scared me. I did not think I could learn in that situation. The medicine rotation was considered the toughest clinical rotation of our second year. It would follow my psychiatry rotation, leaving me ill prepared for the physical rigors of medicine, although perhaps better mentally prepared.

Because I worked every sixth night in the blood bank at Duke to make ends meet financially, I needed to schedule my medicine rotation at Duke rather than the Durham VA Hospital. Osler Ward, the female public ward, was Stead's favorite rounding assignment. I intentionally requested Long Ward, the public male ward, to avoid Dr. Stead.

What followed was an experience in learning that would influence my choice of internal medicine specialty training and, ultimately, rheumatology subspecialty fellowship. I remember the house staff who introduced me to the excitement of clinical medicine. Junior residents Ed Overfield and Dave Treiman were complemented by interns Rich Knazek and Gary Burger. Whether taking care of patients or making forays in the middle of the night to furnish our doctors' office, the experience was stimulating and, while as advertised, incredibly demanding, the final result was fun. There was immediate collegiality; we had a common focus—the best care for our Long Ward patients. The senior attending physicians were kind and patient for an unsophisticated and clinically ignorant student. Dr. Herb Sieker and Dr. Wendell Rosse alternated days making attending rounds for student presentations of new admissions. At the patient's bedside, without notes, the student would make a formal presentation of the history and physical followed by a discussion in the doctor's office and a note written in the chart by the attending physician. This was from 10:00 AM till noon every day except Sunday.

At the same time, Dr. Stead was rounding on Osler Ward. My only contact was an occasional noon conference or Saturday CPC (Clinical Pathological Conference). I remember his lanky arm raised for a question or poignant comment or criticism. What was he doing? He was the past chairman and this was Dr. Wyngaarden's department, wasn't it? At least on Long Ward, I was avoiding him.

However, one morning four weeks into the seven-week rotation, as we were tidying up the doctors' office for teaching rounds, the door opened and Dr. Stead appeared, announcing his substitution on that day rounding for Dr. Sieker. I was scheduled to present and at the sight of Dr. Stead, as sphincters tightened, heart rate increased, and blood pressure rose, I forgot my patient's name and all details of his hospitalization.

Somehow I got through the presentation with only one minor mistake pointed out later in good humor by my resident and interns. I referred to the pulses on top the feet as "dorsal pedalis" rather than "dorsalis pedis" pulses. The patient had a pulmonary embolus (blood clot in the lung) and was doing well as we anticoagulated his blood with heparin. In discussion of the case, I mentioned an article out just that week in the *New England Journal of Medicine* suggesting very high doses of heparin and extreme thinning of the blood. I expressed surprise that Dr. Stead was not aware of the article. I assumed that this icon and godfather of internal medicine knew everything and was up to date on the most recent medical journals.

140

He was kind. "Mr. (note: not Dr.) Wilson, don't teach me something that won't be true two years from now." How could I know if it would still be true? In the book *E. A. Stead, Jr.: What this Patient Needs is a Doctor,* Dr. Stead mentions the frustration of learning something that does not remain valid. Unlearning is twice as hard as learning—my first direct lesson from him. It's reminiscent of the Will Rogers's quote: "It's not what you don't know that will hurt you; it's what you know that ain't so."

Over the next nine years of training, I would encounter Dr. Stead many times. What I learned from my first experience was his demand for honesty and industry. As the physician, you had to put the time and energy in the investigation of your patient. You should know all the test results and details of treatment and response. You might not be able to put together the history, physical, and test findings as diagnostic for congestive heart failure, or Crohn's disease, or Whipple's disease, but he knew the first step was honesty in obtaining the information. The knowledge of diagnosis and treatment would come with time, and, hopefully, wisdom would follow.

The realization of Stead's impact on my training occurred between 1974 and 1976 during our time ironically away from Duke while serving in the Navy at Mayport Naval Station, Jacksonville, Florida (See..."You and Dr. Burton Were Right"). As a General Medical Officer, I had much more free time for reading. During medical school, I felt I could complete about 25 percent of my desired reading. This decreased to about 10 percent during house staff training (internship and residency). It was time to catch up.

In addition to a careful digestion of my *Harrison's Textbook of Internal Medicine,* I began to read a copy of Dr. Stead's book *Just Say for Me.* Dr. Stead would always begin his attending notes after the patient presentation with this introduction, then follow with diagnosis, suggestions or, if he felt the patient's care was not satisfactory, the ultimate criticism: "Just say for me, what this patient needs is a doctor." Ouch.

After pointing out several passages to Sandra, she began reading the book. She made a correct observation: "This is your philosophy of medicine. These are the principles you practice." I realized what many Duke medical students and house officers before and after me had understood. Although we trained in Dr. James B. Wyngaarden's program, so many of the tenets and principles were Dr. Stead's. His influence persisted then and now. Dr. Wyngaarden was kind enough and wise enough to perpetuate the Steadian philosophy in his department.

Did Dr. Stead know this? I believe so. Whenever asked, however, he always demurred saying it was Dr. Wyngaarden's department. Years later, in the early 1980s, while developing my rheumatology practice in Lynchburg, I was serving as a local medical representative to the Medical Society of Virginia. Each year at the annual meeting, there was a reception for Duke Medical School alumni and Dr. Stead came as Duke's representative. I always enjoyed the opportunity to socialize and catch up on Duke. At one reception, I told Dr. Stead, "You know, those of us in training at that time thought it was Wyngaarden's department, but your influence still affected us." No, no. He reassured me that it was Wyngaarden's department, but I believe he was pleased with the observation.

A unique feature of the medicine training program was the connection of authority, responsibility, and ownership (See… "You're the Doc"). As a second year student on the rotation, you were assigned two patients a week for the first three weeks, then three patients a week for the final four weeks. The day or night the patient was admitted, you had to have the results of a chemistry screen, chest x-ray, blood count, EKG, stool for occult blood, and urinalysis (all done by the student or intern) recorded with the handwritten history and physical exam ready for the resident's morning report to the chairman of the department of medicine. Special procedures such as spinal taps, blood cultures, IVs, thoracenteses (drawing fluid out of the chest) were the responsibility of the student or intern. Complicated procedures were taught on a "see one; do one; teach one" method.

The infamous five nights out of seven call schedule applied to students as well as house staff (interns and residents). It assured that the Duke tradition was maintained: you learned

142

medicine by being there. For better or worse this was your patient. You were responsible for knowing all the test results and details of treatment and the patient's course during the hospitalization.

Recognizing the *responsibility* assumed by the intern or student, *authority* was achieved by only following orders written by the patient's intern or student. If a medicine, procedure, or test was to be ordered, the individual responsible for the patient would know it. A consultant could not order a test or treatment until he justified the need for a diagnostic test or treatment with the student or intern—a great teaching method. Authority was earned by taking responsibility and you experienced a sense of *ownership* because no one knew that patient better than you.

Unfortunately, there has been an increasing disconnect between authority and responsibility with the doctor's authority challenged by health insurers, hospital health care systems, and government regulations (See…"You're the Doc" and "I Don't Like That Electric Record"). With that disconnect there is less feeling of ownership of a patient. During my thirty-five years of practice in Lynchburg, I always appreciated hearing a patient tell me: "I'm (insert one: Dr. Craddock's, Dr. Howard's, Dr. McCabe's) patient," or "Dr. (insert one: Craddock, Howard, McCabe) is my doctor." Ownership was felt both ways: physician ownership of the patient and patient ownership of the physician.

Today, the patient may not identify with a particular doctor and vice versa. This is exemplified in the hospitalist movement in most hospitals. The patient may have several different doctors during a hospitalization or even during one day. "Who's your doctor?" may be a difficult question to answer. While I'm told that patients expect and accept this, I'm not convinced they like it. Fewer doctors feel or want ownership of the patient. The attraction for hospitalist and emergency room physicians with fixed hours is the rental of the patient for eight or twelve hours, but not ownership.

So, how did my initial lesson from Dr. Stead work out? Like so many great teachings, it was relevant for the remainder of my practice. The old maxim of not being the first to embrace the new or last to discard the old is still valid in medicine. As I would read the journals, the newest diagnostic procedures and treatments were noted. However, if they were not compatible with my practice experience, I observed them but did not adapt or learn them, and the tincture of time proved or disproved their merit.

I will always remain grateful for the training and preparation I received for the challenges of practice over the years. If someone asks me about my Duke medical education, I proudly tell them it held me in good Stead.

# "YOU'RE CRAZY IF YOU STAY HERE"

Always consider the source. In this case, I was worried. Paul was a role model: a Sigma Nu fraternity brother two years my senior, a hard worker as a Duke undergraduate student, a good athlete, and he was no crybaby. He delivered this advice at 2:00 AM one spring morning toward the end of my third year of medical school.

Unusual time for such a caveat? We were meeting at the Blood Bank where I worked every sixth night during med school as the technician typing and crossing for emergency transfusion needs. Paul was picking up three units of blood for a patient with a bleeding ulcer. He was in the midst of his internal medicine internship, and he was exhausted. On the public wards of Osler, Long, and Strudwick, the intern was on call five nights out of seven. He or she carried a beeper and could go home as soon as the work was done. "Work done" was an oxymoron. If the intern got home before 1:00 AM, he was lucky and felt that he would be extra refreshed when returning at 7:00 the next morning.

Paul knew I was planning to do an internal medicine internship. When he spoke, I listened. And every time we passed in the hospital, Paul repeated this warning. But I noticed something. Paul was becoming an excellent doctor.

Other interns shared sobering stories regarding the demands of the internship year. Dr. Jim Bass recalled his first rotation at the Durham VA Hospital. He was assigned to 7B floor, which was split half medicine, half neurology. Jim was the only intern sharing ward duties with one resident. The VA was not air conditioned so by the end of the first day (July 1, 1971), Jim's crisp starched white intern jacket and underlying tie and shirt were abandoned—dressed down to his sweaty T-shirt.

He was determined to do a full workup on every old patient he was picking up, as well as the new admissions. By the time his evening off came around three days later, he had not left the hospital. The resident demanded that he go home. When he got home at 7:00 that evening his wife had dinner waiting. After eating, Jim put his feet up and the next thing he knew his wife was shaking his shoulders. "That's nice," he thought, "she's waking me up to go to bed." But, surprise! His spouse shook him awake, delivering heartbreaking news, "Honey, wake up, it's morning. Time to go back to the hospital." Jim confided that on the drive back to the hospital he couldn't help it— tears were rolling involuntarily down both cheeks.

Next year, the Duke Medical School class of 1972 would simultaneously learn our internship fates one day in March— National Match Day. This was a new system to hopefully elimi- nate some of the confusion as med school graduates tried to secure post-graduate training positions. Interviews were held during the fall and winter. The med student and the training pro- gram rated their choices. For example, if Duke internal medi- cine was your first choice but they rated you at a level three, you might not match there, but if the University of Pittsburgh School of Medicine rated you #1 and you rated them #2, a match might be made.

During my clinical rotations, I was impressed with several teaching house staff and Duke med school faculty who were inbred like me. Inbred? It meant you had been an undergradu- ate at Duke, went to Duke Med School, and stayed on for post- graduate training. Some of the residents in orthopedics, neuro- surgery, and cardiovascular surgery had been at Duke for fifteen to twenty years. The attitude was "Don't go somewhere else, unless you can go somewhere better."

There were few training programs in internal medicine better than Duke. So in the fall of my senior year in med school, I was flattered to get a call to make an appointment to see Dr. Grace Kirby. She oversaw the medical internship program. Dr. Kirby had been the first female chief resident in medicine at Duke. While she was a member of the rheumatology depart- ment, she was best known for her role as medical intern orga- nizer.

Others had the same attitude as Paul regarding the medical internship. The med school yearbook had a picture of Dr. Kirby looking over internship applications with the caption, "Who will join the Ship of Fools this year?" So I was certainly forewarned when I showed up for my appointment. Dr. Kirby said that based on my record, they wanted to offer me a medical internship position. If I would make Duke my first choice, they would rate me as a first choice and the match would be guaranteed. I did express some concerns about the rigors of the internship and may have mentioned Paul's caveat. Would I be able to handle the work load? Dr. Kirby assured me that I could do the work and promised me that I would learn a level of efficiency I couldn't imagine. I accepted the offer and they kept their promise. My contract was simple. "The undersigned will be on call to the Department of Medicine from July 1, 1972 until June 30, 1973, for $7,000.00."

So how did things work out? I never worked harder nor had more fun. In medical education, there is a theory that the physician you become is a reflection of your training. I believe that is true. My training really started in the fall of 1969 (See... "Don't Teach Me Something That Won't Be True Two Years From Now"), with formal Duke training ending in July 1979, and the seeds for continuing medical education firmly planted. So, in spite of Paul's warning, I'm glad I stayed and I'm reminded of Paul Simon's song, "Still Crazy After All These Years."

# "I HAVE A NEW TITLE"
## (How the Patient Affects a Disease— Sjögren's Syndrome)

While a doctor is always concerned about the way a disease affects his patient, on a rare occasion he has the joy of witnessing how an exceptional patient affects a disease. Katherine Morland Hammitt's new title is Vice President of Medical and Scientific Affairs for the Sjögren's Syndrome Foundation. In this capacity, she oversees key research and medical initiatives that will increase knowledge about Sjögren's Syndrome, resulting in improved treatment and management of the disease.

Quite a journey to this new position since her initial visit to my office on November 11, 1984, presenting as a worried thirty-two-year-old mother of a one and a half-year-old daughter. She received a call Friday evening from a University of Virginia (UVa) resident physician with the news that she was diagnosed with Sjögren's Syndrome. Of more concern was the possibility of a rare complication related to the disease. A shadow on her chest x-ray could represent lymphoma (a form of lymph node cancer). She would need a chest CT scan to clarify the possibility, but this could not be scheduled for several months at UVa. The resident told Kathy that a delay in obtaining the test would not matter since, if lymphoma was present, there was no effective treatment. Not very reassuring; no wonder she was worried.

We were able to schedule the CT scan right away. It showed an enlarged area in the middle part of the chest—the mediastinum. Over the next few months Kathy, her family, and I, as her new rheumatologist, worried about this mediastinal mass on the CT scan. Did we need to proceed with chest surgery to biopsy this area? Not a simple operation. We benefited from the wisdom of our thoracic surgeon, Dr. Jensie Teague, and opted for watchful waiting. Surgery was not performed then and, thankfully, never in the future.

148

At this time, Kathy began learning everything about Sjögren's. Like so many Sjögren's patients, there had been a long delay in her diagnosis. As a chronic autoimmune disease of protean manifestations, Sjögren's often presents signs and symptoms such as sicca (dry eyes and dry mouth), parotid swelling, fatigue, arthralgias, and dental problems for years before the diagnosis is made. For a brief time, I knew more about Sjögren's Syndrome and autoimmune diseases than my patient. This changed quickly, however, as she studied the disease and became actively involved in the organization.

What does an activist patient do? Like Kathy, he or she becomes involved at several levels. She has served the Sjögren's Syndrome Foundation in many capacities: President, interim Executive Director, Director of Research Development and Public Policy, and her current position. As editor of *The Sjögren's Quarterly*, she directs information to physicians as well as patients. She was an associate editor for *The Sjögren's Book*, 4th edition and co-authored Chapter 34 "Disability and Sjögren's."

As a patient, she recognized the dearth of practical information for people suffering with Sjögren's. In 2003, *The Sjögren's Syndrome Survival Guide* co-authored by Kathy and Teri Rumpf (a clinical psychologist and Sjögren's patient) was published and remains an important aid for all patients.

She attends national and international meetings related to Sjögren's Syndrome. Many trips to Washington, D.C. were made advocating for Sjögren's awareness and research support at the national level. She even produced a bumper sticker for the rheumatologist as an endangered species. Not surprisingly, this combination of intelligence and industry has resulted in a true Sjögren's expert, far more knowledgeable than most physicians and rheumatologists (myself included).

Kathy's activist journey has been exceptional. Her family background includes physician grandfathers, a college professor father, and mother, Margaret Morland, who was the poet laureate of Virginia. Impressive inherited genes, I believe, have been a factor as she's followed this path from self-education to prominence at the national and international level. She continues to enhance the current understanding of Sjögren's Syndrome and influence future directions for research and treatment.

While few patients could affect their diseases to a similar degree, contributions to research, participation in support groups and activities, such as sponsored walks and health fairs, are all important. A favorite scripture of mine is Mark 14:8 (The Anointing at Bethany) when Jesus says, "She has done what she could..." If a patient is doing all they can at any level, they are an activist affecting their disease and share a new title with Kathy—"Hero" or "Heroine."

# "THANKS"
## (The Doctor Patient)

February 21, 2011. I was in no position to receive grati-
tude. It was my wife's birthday and instead of celebrating her
long awaited cruise to Panama, I was in pre-op getting ready
for Dr. Robert Sydnor to replace my right hip. I might have expected a sarcastic "Thanks a lot," from Sandra after cancelling
the cruise, but this thanks came from my anesthesiologist.

"For what?" We had already completed my orientation
interview deciding on general anesthesia. He had gone on to
other pre-op patients, my IV was started, senses were blissfully
numbing out with drowsiness settling in, but he returned...
"Thanks for not playing the doctor card."

Some of the staff in pre-op had recognized me in spite of
hospital gown, footies, no glasses, and a hair net qualifying me
for surgery or food service work. When they asked the anesthesiologist about "Dr. Wilson," he came back. I appreciated the
courtesy visit, but he did not have to worry about any expectations of special "doctor" care.

While I don't like being on the receiving end of medical
treatment, when I'm a patient, that's it. I'm not "Dr." patient;
I'm the simplest "Average Joe" patient. As I woke up post-op in
my room, I was introduced to my patient aide. James was an
African American, probably in his mid-fifties. His first words
were, "You're a doctor, huh?" It was more of a declaration than
a question. "Yes," I admitted, "but here I'm just a patient." I
think James's attitude was wait and see. His care was excellent.

Over the next two days, James was on the morning shift
so we interacted at several levels: assistance to the bathroom,
bathing, meals, and preparation for Joint Camp activities. He
called me "Doc." Like many long-standing patients or even
with my extended family office staff (See... "You Have the Best

Office"), they're more comfortable with the familiar "Doc" than "Jeff."

On the morning of discharge, James said, "You know, Doc, you smell pretty good." When someone comments favorably on my attire or scent, I have to credit my family. Sandra and daughters, Elizabeth and Melissa, jointly pick out shirts and ties, while Melissa personally Christmas gifts my annual supply of Polo cologne. "Must be the Polo," I explained. "I may not end the day smelling good, but I start out smelling great. You smell good, too, James. What're you wearing?"

Guess what? James used Polo as well. When Sandra arrived to take me home, I couldn't wait to tell her. With James in the room helping us gather my belongings, I told her James and I were Polo brothers. She loved the coincidence of fraternal bonding by Polo.

As I headed down the hall toward the elevators, James's last words were, "You know, Doc, you're all right."

A welcomed accolade. And a patient, not a doctor, went home.

# "I DON'T DRINK THAT MUCH"

## (The Iron Man—Hemochromatosis)

My sixty-two-year-old patient, F. E., was angry and depressed. His primary care physician found abnormal liver blood
tests on his yearly check-up and told F. E., it was probably from
excess alcohol intake. In plain language, "You're drinking too
much and it's hurting your liver."

The metric for "drinking too much" varies from patient
to patient and doctor to doctor. The most human and humane
measure of "too much" is the person who has one more drink
than I do. On the other hand, an accurate social history of alcohol use is open to interpretation. "What sort of alcohol? Hard
liquor, beer, wine? Every night? How many drinks each week or
night? Ever interfere with your work or driving?"

F. E. was not a teetotaler. Before the abnormal blood tests
were discovered, he had a beer each night, occasional glass of
wine when eating dinner out at a restaurant, and only a rare
cocktail. I had to agree with his evaluation, "I don't drink that
much." Nevertheless, he stopped all forms of alcohol but, after
three months of abstinence, liver function tests were more abnormal, and now he had arthritis. No wonder he was angry and
depressed when he came for his rheumatology evaluation.

His workup was notable for family history of a brother with
heart failure who required a heart transplant, but no family history of rheumatoid arthritis. A review of medical records and referral note from his primary doctor revealed moderate elevation
of liver function tests and a slightly high glucose (sugar) level.
His physician had noted some darkening of his skin, which he
attributed to liver disease.

The diagnostic clue came in examining his hands. F. E.
was bothered with pain in all of his fingers, but notably in the
knuckles at the base of the fingers (MCP—metacarpophalan-

geal joints). There was bony swelling of the joints, but no soft tissue swelling to suggest RA (rheumatoid arthritis). X-rays of the hands showed OA (osteoarthritis) changes and calcification in some joint cartilages.

OA in this unusual location alerts the rheumatologist to two conditions. Acromegaly—a tumor of the pituitary gland may cause this (See..."This Headache Is Different"), but the combination of skin hyperpigmentation, elevated blood sugar, OA changes on x-ray with probable chondrocalcinosis (calcium in the cartilages) in MCP joints, and family history of heart disease suggested a diagnosis of hemochromatosis sometimes referred to as "Bronze diabetes."

This is an inherited disorder in which iron accumulates in various organs. F. E.'s diagnosis was suggested by abnormal iron blood tests and confirmed by a liver biopsy. Elevated serum iron level with decreased total iron binding capacity (TIBC) and elevated ferritin level were compatible with iron overload found in the liver biopsy.

Treatment included frequent phlebotomy to decrease iron stores. Family members were referred for genetic testing. His arthritis stabilized, but did not go away with phlebotomy. It was controlled with naproxen. Liver function blood tests improved and he did not progress on to heart failure. Depression and anger cleared when alcoholic liver disease was ruled out, but F. E. remained a teetotaler.

Note: My patient's identity is protected by using the initials F. E. Remember your Periodic Table in chemistry class? Fe is the designation for iron. Appropriate for my Iron Man. Sorry, "my bad"—rheumatologist humor.

# "MY DOCTOR THINKS I HAVE LUPUS"
## (Alpha Gal Tick Disease)

My eighty-three-year-old patient (M. P.) gave up an appointment time so her daughter, Jill, could be seen sooner for my rheumatology evaluation. Jill was a fifty-five-year-old white female followed by dermatologist, Dr. Grace Newton, for the problem of recurrent hives. A biopsy revealed urticarial vasculitis, a condition usually associated with lupus. Concerns that Jill might have this uncommon presentation of lupus prompted the rheumatology referral. But the ANA (Antinuclear Antibody) test was negative, and while rheumatologists see many false positive tests, a negative ANA really rules out lupus 99+ percent of the time.

Jill lived in a rural setting with abundant tick exposure and occasional bites, but no history of any severe rash or reaction around a specific bite. The usual tick panel blood test was negative for Lyme disease, ehrlichiosis, babesiosis, and Rocky Mountain Spotted Fever, but because of the urticarial (hive) component, I checked the alpha gal IgE test which was positive at 14.00 kU/L (normal <0.35). She denied any mammalian meat intolerance, but, like so many of our patients, irritable bowel symptoms had caused her to modify her diet toward more of a fish, chicken, and vegetable menu.

There are many unique things about practicing in Lynchburg and our Central Virginia area, especially for more than three decades. Long term relationships developed with patients and their families. MP reminded me that I had seen Jill more than eight years earlier in consultation at Virginia Baptist Hospital with the same question—could she have lupus? She was bothered with essentially a giant hive on her right arm. Lupus was ruled out with negative blood tests (including the ANA test) and the absence of diagnostic criteria for lupus except the skin changes. I think she had alpha gal tick disease at that time, before we even knew it existed.

Her mother (M. P.) was followed in my office for over twenty years, taking methotrexate and hydroxychloroquine for a chronic inflammatory arthritis associated with an atypical rash on her fingers. Considering similar rural background and tick population exposure, I checked the alpha gal IgE test on M. P., and guess what? Positive at 3.18 kU/L. She likewise had no marked mammalian meat sensitivity.

These findings stimulated my interest in alpha gal tick disease during the last fifteen months of my rheumatology practice from September 2013 through December 15, 2014. I added the alpha gal IgE blood test whenever there was a question of tick exposure related to the patient's symptoms. Out of more than 200 patients tested, the routine tick panels detected one case of Lyme disease, two cases of ehrilichiosis, and one case of Rocky Mountain Spotted Fever. One hundred forty-seven patients had (+) blood tests for alpha gal.

Only eleven of these patients had known mammalian meat sensitivity, with symptoms varying from urticaria to angioedema, but no anaphylaxis episodes. Interestingly, Jill called several weeks after her (+) alpha gal test noting a flare of hives after eating potatoes! But those potatoes had spent the day in a crock pot with a beef pot roast, so plenty of mammalian meat exposure.

The majority of patients had no history of typical mammalian meat sensitivity and instead presented with a mixed group of signs and symptoms. Like Lyme disease, alpha gal tick disease is a disorder with protean manifestations including: varied rashes, paresthesias (numbness or tingling), sciatica, carpal tunnel syndrome, abdominal pain, diarrhea, asthma, arthralgias, myalgias, and inflammatory arthritis.

In treating my alpha gal (+) patients, I asked them to follow a mammalian meat restricted diet for six weeks. Many patients reported improvement in joint symptoms, skin rash, paresthesias, and asthma. One family was most interesting. Father, son, and daughter were all (+) for alpha gal. The father and son had the highest levels found among my patients, > 100 kU/L. They were cattle ranchers, avid beef eaters, and none had classic symptoms of mammalian meat allergy. However, after six weeks on the restricted diet, arthritis was improved in all three, and the seventy-eight-year-old father had noticed that belly pain waking him for years in the middle of the night was gone. I suspect he had a gastrointestinal manifestation of his alpha gal tick disease causing abdominal pain hours after eating his evening meal. I had several other alpha gal tick disease patients with gastrointestinal symptoms including abdominal pain with or without diarrhea after a meal containing mammalian meat. A nurse who had previously worked at our office was hospitalized three times with abdominal pain before they diagnosed alpha gal tick disease.

Sometimes diet instruction was difficult. One alpha gal (+) patient was an avid hunter. After the usual caveat to avoid beef, pork, and lamb, he had questions. "What about... (he began a list, countering my answer "No, mammal" with another choice each time) ...deer, rabbit, squirrel, bison, bear, possum?" "No, no, no; mammal, mammal, mammal. Remember ninth grade biology class?" No patient asked about it, but I wonder about whale meat. A question I'll save for my first Eskimo patient.

While many patients improved with diet restriction, if there was no response or only partial improvement, the patient was treated with doxycycline following the usual Lyme disease protocol. Just like Lyme tick disease, some patients improved with antibiotics with or without diet restriction. I suspect, like Jill's mother, some alpha gal tick disease patients may have a chronic inflammatory arthritis requiring treatment regimens similar to therapies used for rheumatoid arthritis.

So Jill did not have lupus. Instead, she had the most prevalent tick disease in our area and probably in the entire Southeast. The possibility of alpha gal tick disease needs to be considered by primary care providers, dermatologists, neurologists, gastroenterologists, and rheumatologists whenever the possibility of a tick related disease is part of the differential diagnosis. It requires a specific test (alpha gal IgE test) which is *not* part of the tick panel available through commercial labs. Until our health care providers become more aware of alpha gal tick disease as more than an allergic reaction, the most common tick disease will also remain the most underdiagnosed.

# "SHOULDN'T I GO HOME?"

## (Doctor on Call)

My phone rang at 1:00 AM. The answering service asked me to call the number for a ward at the Training School. That's unusual, I thought. I had seen a few of their patients in consultation, but was never contacted this late at night. I knew some of our Lynchburg Family Practice residents were moonlighting at CVTC. Maybe one of them had a problem or question. But the ward nurse who answered the phone was the patient of a physician I shared call with.

"Doctor Wilson, I'm a diabetic and I forgot to take my insulin. My sugar's high, shouldn't I go home?"

Even as a young physician, being awakened out of sleep in the middle of the night leaves your senses and reasoning a little muddled. When I was a medical intern, we lived in a tiny apartment on Watts Street in Durham with one phone in the hall outside the bedroom. I arrived home around 1:30 AM one night, going into a deep sleep as soon as my head hit the pillow. Sandra had gone to bed hours earlier.

When the phone rang at 3:00 AM, I heard Sandra answering the call, "He's not here. I think he's still at the hospital." She didn't even know I was in bed beside her! "Wait, wait, Sandra, I'm here." She handed off the phone. She was probably just in the twilight of returning to sleep when she heard me say, "I'm thinking, I'm thinking." I had fallen asleep leaning against the wall, phone pressed against my ear. The nurse had explained that my diabetic patient was having a low blood sugar episode but after two minutes of silence, she summoned me again, "Doctor Wilson, Doctor Wilson! Are you okay!?" The honest response would be, "I'm dog tired and fell asleep holding the phone," but "I'm thinking, I'm thinking" seemed more professional. Some IV glucose and readjustment of insulin took care of the patient and I returned to sleep in a reclining rather than standing position.

One night in the Virginia Baptist MICU (Medical Intensive Care Unit), I realized I was not alone in sleep deprived mentation problems. It was around 2:00 AM, I was transferring one of my patients to the MICU (See..."He's Gone") and a nurse was chuckling as she hung up the phone. "I just called Dr. Bendall about some labs on his patient. He told me to give him a box of chocolates and call back in the morning." Well, probably better than "take two aspirin and call me in the morning" or "I'm thinking, I'm thinking."

But at this late hour, something about the CVTC call didn't seem right. I remember one of the residents telling me that when moonlighting, they spent more time handling staff sick call than tending to patients. I asked the nurse what time she realized she'd missed her evening insulin. I was surprised and peeved when she said at 9:00 PM. "And you waited till 1:00 AM to call?"

Well, she was busy till she got to work. Go home? Oh, no. There couldn't be a better place to get her sugar back under control than right there among fellow nurses in the hospital setting. While this meant being called every two hours as I adjusted her insulin, I thought it was worth it. "And incidentally, let me be sure to get your name right." "Why? Because I'm going to send you a bill for this."

She was incensed. "My regular doctor doesn't charge me for medical advice over the phone." "Well, I'll tell you what," I responded, "call your lawyer at two in the morning and see if you get free legal advice. If he doesn't charge you, I won't either."

Her diabetes was controlled after several calls that night, she received a bill, and she never called me in the middle of the night again.

# "YOU'RE NEVER GOING TO GET A REAL JOB, ARE YOU?"

## (Medical Knowledge Explosion)

Harsh words from your own mother. Followed by an almost accusatory observation, "You're a professional student." Mom's comments were understandable. Our immediate relatives included the families of her two sisters. Out of five male cousins and the three pairs of parents, there were three college graduates. Mother (June Hartman Wilson) graduated from Marshall College (class of 1937), cousin Mike Bush from WVU (West Virginia University 1967), and I finished my undergraduate degree at Duke in 1968. No one else had gone on to medical school or any formal post-graduate education.

With med school graduation two months away, members of our class eagerly awaited "The Match." On one designated day in March, graduating seniors at all med schools would learn where they would spend their first year of post-graduate training (See…"You're Crazy If You Stay Here"). I would begin my internship at Duke in the medicine department July 1972.

According to Mom, at that time, I could begin practice in West Virginia without completing an internship. Surely, after four years of medical school you were ready to practice; you must know everything. I explained that I needed more post graduate education provided by the internship year. When I stayed for junior residency the next year, she again reminded me that I could set up practice in West Virginia without further training.

Two years in the Navy at Mayport, Florida, were followed by a return to Duke for the senior residency year. When I announced that I wanted to stay for a two-year fellowship in rheumatology, my mother couldn't contain herself, "You're never going to get a real job, are you? You're a professional student."

In reality, I believe she felt that if I didn't know everything by then I must be a little slow.

Over the years, after settling in Lynchburg and starting my rheumatology practice, Mom's visits, and later establishing her residency here, reassured her that I had finally gotten a "real" job. But she was right about one thing. I had become a professional student, and I believe that was the intent of our Duke training—learning to learn.

My wife laughs as I subscribe to and study each edition of the MKSAP (Medical Knowledge Self-Assessment Program). This is produced about every two years and serves as an example of the exponential increase in medical knowledge. I took every edition through MKSAP #16, which says a little about my age and time in practice. MKSAP #1 came out while I was in house staff training (1972). In about 120 pages, it covered all the general and subspecialty areas of internal medicine. It was full of up-to-date information and what we called "pearls" in practice—signs or symptoms that provided clues for diagnosis and treatment of difficult or confusing cases. It was excellent preparation for internal medicine board certification at that time and subsequent editions have been a great source for continuing medical education over the years. As you might guess, to cover the advances in the area of internal medicine alone, MKSAP has expanded to twelve separate booklets (over 1000 pages) including general medicine and all the subspecialty areas. Each section is about the same size as the total original MKSAP #1 with basic text of 120 to 150 pages, followed by a similar number of pages, including clinical presentation quizzes and excellent discussion of the cases.

Keeping up to date is difficult even in a single subspecialty. Kudos to my primary care physician friends who are coordinating care for the entire patient. One evening at the Free Clinic I was asked by an attending endocrinologist which journals I regularly reviewed. The list included the following: *New England Journal of Medicine; Annals of Internal Medicine; Journal of the American Medical Association; American Journal of Medicine; Mayo Clinic Proceedings; Arthritis & Rheumatism;*

various newsletters—AMA *News, The Rheumatologist, Internal Medicine News, Rheumatology News.*

Managing the material from so many journals can be a challenge. Over forty years ago, I became a tearer (not a terror). Articles of interest would be cut out using an old scalpel and categorized to fit in my file cabinet. After years of collecting articles, the cabinet should be bursting at its seams. But, no. For every article added, one was removed. Usually, in each folder there would be an out-of-date paper, perhaps a treatment or diagnostic test no longer proven effective. However, some articles were retained as classics of rheumatology. I shared my files with Family Practice residents, nurse practitioners, and medical students. I remember the response of a family practice resident during a rheumatology rotation in the fall 2001 when I showed her the article "Arteritis of the Aged (Giant Cell Arteritis) and Fever of Unexplained Origin" from the March 1976 *American Journal of Medicine.* "Why, Dr. Wilson, that's the year I was born." It made me feel like a classic.

I believe the government could learn something from my filing system. No new law is added unless an old, extant one is eliminated. I remember an exchange between Sam Donaldson and George Will years ago on "Meet the Press." Donaldson was berating the Republicans for stopping Congress from doing its work. George Will asked what that work was. "You know. Making laws." George's reply was a question, "Oh, is there a shortage of laws in our country?" Obviously not. Likewise, the Federal Registry expanding yearly by more than 25,000 pages has become inane, too large and unusable. I would suggest that at the beginning of the newly elected Congress, instead of reading the Constitution, read the Federal Registry and eliminate the unintelligible and useless material. Nancy Pelosi set a worrisome precedent with the Affordable Care Act. Just vote it into law and you can read it later. Some members of Congress may have eventually read it, but I wonder if anyone understands it.

With the exponential increase in medical knowledge, I never felt up to date. The more I learned, the more aware I became of my ignorance and deficiencies. But maybe that's the nature of a professional student. While I proved Mom wrong as far as getting a real job, her claim that I was a professional student was accurate. No excuses; may it continue.

# "THAT'S WHAT YOU TOLD ME TO DO, DOC"

## ("SOS" Doctor in Training)

We always remember our first, don't we? R. H. was my first patient. This seventy-eight-year-old African American farmer was admitted to the Long Ward medical service (See..."Don't Teach Me Something That Won't Be True Two Years From Now") for problems of back pain and anemia. Admission labs and x-rays were obtained.

The work-up of anemia always requires ruling out any gastrointestinal blood loss, frequently a sign of colon cancer. This would entail checking serial stool samples for occult blood. I instructed R. H. to save any stool samples for testing.

Over the next week, we discovered that R. H. had multiple myeloma, most likely the cause of his back pain and anemia. One of our attending senior physicians, Dr. Wendell Rosse, was a hematologist. He would be ideal for my medical student presentation on teaching rounds. Our two interns, my two fellow medical students, Dr. Rosse, and I gathered at the bedside. I began with the patient profile: "Mr. R. H. is a seventy-eight-year-old married farmer from Fayetteville..." But I suddenly stopped, gagging as I was overcome by a terrible odor.

Good heavens, what's that smell! R. H. was on the open ward with sixteen beds separated only by hanging curtains and a shared bedside cabinet. The smell of old poop wafted in the air. It did not require great detective work to track down the source. I followed my nose to the bedside cabinet. When I opened the door there were six stool samples wrapped in toilet paper on a shelf. "R. H., what's this?" I asked. "What are these stool samples doing in here?"

"That's what you told me to do, Doc." R. H. was just following my instructions—my incomplete instructions. What I meant was to collect a small stool sample after each bowel movement, place it in a specimen cup, put a lid on the cup, and give it to me or the nurse. It would stay in the lab refrigerator until I tested it for occult blood and discarded the specimen.

As I collected the week-old seasoned specimens and performed the lab tests, I learned some valuable lessons for a doctor in training. You can't be too careful or detailed in your instructions to a patient. Murphy's Law is always in force. Anticipation of misunderstanding or foul-ups can avoid problems, and avoidance is definitely better than correction—especially when dealing with an "SOS"—"Save Our Stool."

# "YOU MUST NOT BE MUCH OF A RHEUMATOLOGIST"

## (Age and the Doctor/Patient Fool)

My patient, J. C., was kidding—I think. I had just informed him that I would be out of the office for six weeks recovering from spinal stenosis surgery scheduled November 20, 2012. He remembered that my right hip was replaced in 2010 (See… "Thanks—The Doctor Patient"). The most common form of arthritis—wear and tear, degenerative, osteoarthritis—was behind the surgeries. If the rheumatologist couldn't take care of his own common form of arthritis, he "must not be much of a rheumatologist."

J. C. understood my explanation. While our medicines and modalities, such as physical therapy, might slow down the wear and tear, there was something I couldn't do. Stop time or turn back the clock (See…"I Know What's Wrong"). As long as we live, we'll be wearing down. I liked the attitude of our patients who say they'd rather wear out than rust out. My goal for all the arthritis patients was to be able to do what you want to do as well as what you need to do. As a patient on the receiving end of arthritis care, I realized the modification of this philosophy—the shift more toward need than want and the change in my bucket list. I have given up the chance to play point guard for the Duke basketball team and replaced that with the goal of beating my twelve-year-old grandson, Campbell, one more time in a game of H-O-R-S-E.

I could probably destroy all of J. C.'s confidence in his rheumatologist by relating my saga arriving at the diagnosis of Parkinson's disease. Most simply stated, I reaffirmed the maxim: the doctor who had himself as a patient, has a fool for a patient, and a fool for a doctor. Amen.

167

For a year following surgery, while the severe, limiting pain of spinal stenosis was gone, I never could pick up my walking pace. I always fell behind any walking group. I attributed slow gait, mild imbalance, and a slight left foot drop to residuals of the spinal stenosis. All of these were improved with a course of physical therapy.

Walking was my main exercise and next I noticed my left arm was not swinging normally. There was no way to attribute this to back surgery. The doctor/patient fool had a differential of possible neck spinal stenosis causing the left arm symptoms, while post-spinal stenosis back surgery still related to ambulation problems. In medicine, we always try to tie things together in a single diagnosis. I decided I had a slow growing brain tumor (probably a meningioma), which had gradually enlarged from affecting left leg movement to now involving the left arm as well.

I scheduled an appointment with Dr. John Gordon Burch in Roanoke. Gordon had been on the neurology staff at Duke and the Durham VA Hospital when I was a student and house officer. He had been my primary source of clinical neurology education. At the July 28, 2014, appointment, the doctor/patient fool's diagnosis of a brain tumor was replaced with Parkinson's disease.

I was embarrassed as much as surprised, even though the disease was early with mild symptoms. Each year in my practice, I would diagnose Parkinson's disease in one or two patients. Usually, features of resting pill rolling tremor of one hand, jerky passive extension of forearm (cog-wheeling), decreased blinking, and forward walking with short steps almost falling (festinating gait) were tip-offs—confirmed by a neurology referral. So while J. C. thought I must not be much of a rheumatologist, apparently I was even less of a neurologist.

As I drove home from Roanoke on that summer afternoon, a fool patient was dismissed from a fool doctor's practice. But don't tell J. C.

# "MY DAUGHTER'S BURNING UP"

## (Juvenile Arthritis)

Cassie's mom was calling about her daughter's fever of 104 degrees. Frankly, I didn't know what more we could do. Cassie was discharged only two days earlier from the pediatric ward at Virginia Baptist Hospital. Twelve aspirin a day, 20 mg of prednisone twice a day, and six extra strength acetaminophen daily should control any fever. Would we need cooling baths or even a cooling blanket and readmission to the hospital?

Arthritis in children just doesn't seem fair. In 1985 when I first began caring for Cassie, there were no pediatric rheumatologists then or now in Lynchburg. UVa had two excellent, busy pediatric rheumatologists—Dr. Richard Kessler and Dr. Frank Saulsbury (both since retired). Dr. Harry Gewanter was the pediatric rheumatologist in Richmond (still practicing in 2016).

In my rheumatology fellowship, I received pediatric training from Dr. Deborah Kredich. She provided not only knowledge, but molded your perception and attitude about the juvenile arthritis patient. In describing a case or writing a note she always began, "This beautiful child..." You realized it was a privilege to see and treat the child. It was an opportunity to intervene in a way that might make a difference for the rest of their lives. It was a special responsibility and some of the cases like Cassie's were tough.

Cassie was admitted to the hospital by her pediatrician for an FUO—"Fever of Unknown Origin." Just back from summer camp in North Carolina, she had diffuse aches, fever, mild rash, and chest pain. Rocky Mountain Spotted Fever was suspect, but all tests for tick or other infectious processes were negative. The fever, elevated WBC (white blood count), and high sedimentation rate (103 mm/hr—normal <10mm/hr) were signs of an inflammatory disorder—Systemic Onset JRA (Juvenile Rheumatoid Arthritis).

The initial treatments were unsuccessful and gold shots were tried as a hopeful remittive agent. There was no response. I hospitalized Cassie several times for intravenous steroids and parenteral pain meds. Suggestions solicited from my pediatric rheumatology colleagues included a trial of intravenous gammaglobulin. The insurance company balked; it was experimental, unproven. True, but we were desperate. With no insurance coverage, it would cost the family approximately the cost of a new Mercedes every six weeks. No way.

Meanwhile, over the next year, Cassie experienced the problems of uncontrolled inflammation and side effects of prednisone. She had been an athlete on volleyball and track teams and was entering the highs and lows of teenage life. The inflammation fatigued her. There was no energy for sports, shopping trips to the mall with girlfriends, and eventually she had to be home schooled. Cushingoid side effects appeared with prednisone causing a moon face and thinning hair, mild acne, and weakness in her limbs as weight shifted to face and trunk. Remember your teenage years? Was there ever a time you were more self-conscious of appearance? Cassie was being robbed of her youth. What more could we do?

Rheumatology is a small field. There are probably less than one-tenth the number of rheumatologists compared with cardiologists. We run into each other at national and regional meetings, and in reading the journals you become familiar with academic rheumatologists and their research. An article at about that time in *Arthritis & Rheumatism* by Dr. David Brewer discussed the use of methotrexate in JRA. We were just beginning to use it in adult arthritis patients (See…"I'm Not Taking That Damned Cancer Medicine"). I called Dr. Brewer and with some guidance on dosing and treatment regimen, I started Cassie on oral methotrexate.

But, no response. We still could not control the inflammation and taper her prednisone. We boosted her oral methotrexate to maximal doses of 25 mg weekly. At this time, the academics in oncology and rheumatology felt that the bioavailability of methotrexate was the same whether given orally by pill, orally by liquid, or parenterally by shot. But I wondered, with all this systemic illness, maybe she somehow wasn't absorbing the methotrexate. We started giving the methotrexate by weekly subcutaneous or intramuscular injection.

It worked. Cassie and her family were people of great faith and patience. Those may have been factors. Interestingly, years later, the academic rheumatology researchers published evidence that parenteral methotrexate was more effective. Glad we didn't wait for them to discover this. For whatever reason: faith, injectable methotrexate, the disease burning out—it was cause to celebrate.

Over the next year, the JRA went into complete remission. Steroids were tapered off and all the unpleasant side effects resolved. She went back to school and activities. Within another six months, Cassie was tapered off methotrexate and all arthritis meds. Over the next decade, she graduated from college, married, and had two children.

Debbie Kredich assisted with another patient (D. S.) presenting as a nine-year-old boy with systemic JRA. Fever, pain, and WBC over 36,000 caused us concern of possible leukemia. I transferred D. S. to Duke on Debbie's service. Leukemia was ruled out and therapies begun. D. S. never achieved the hoped for remission. He had continued arthritis activity as an adult. Like Cassie, however, he married and the family includes one daughter. His faith and spirit remained undaunted as I followed him over thirty years.

Dr. Deborah Kredich passed away from breast cancer over ten years ago. In addition to her contributions in pediatric rheumatology, Debbie was an advocate for women in medicine. I think she would be proud to see how these two "beautiful children" turned into "beautiful adults." They serve as a local Lynchburg legacy to a "beautiful" pediatric rheumatologist.

I am reminded of the importance of pediatric rheumatology by the line "The Child is the father of the Man" from William Wordsworth's poem "My Heart Leaps Up."

## My Heart Leaps Up

My heart leaps up when I behold
A rainbow in the sky:
So was it when my life began;
So is it now I am a man;
So be it when I shall grow old,
Or let me die!
The Child is the father of the Man;
I could wish my days to be
Bound each to each by natural piety.

# "DIDN'T YOU USED TO BE A DOCTOR?"

During my last year in practice (2014), at a patient's final appointment, I reminded each one that Lynchburg is a small place and I expected to run into them at the grocery store, movies, restaurants—really anywhere in our community. I looked forward to it, and invited them to say *hi*. But outside the office setting, without a long white lab coat and stethoscope, patients sometimes had trouble recognizing me in civilian attire. Usually the question was, "Aren't you Dr. Wilson?" I would answer, "Yes, unless I shaved the wrong guy this morning."

Today's query, "Didn't you used to be a doctor?" came from the daughter of a long-time patient. "Yes, I was your mom's doctor. Give her my regards."

While she really meant, "Aren't you Dr. Wilson?" her question started me to thinking. When does a physician stop being a doctor? When you no longer have an office with scheduled appointments? When you have retired? Most of us during our active practice lives made time for Lynchburg Family Practice Residents, occasional medical students, and a few Nurse Practitioners in training to spend month-long rotations with us. That ended when the office closed. Had I ceased being a doctor?

I would suggest when a physician no longer impacts a community's health, he or she has stopped being a doctor. Missionary and Free Clinic work helps maintain the traditional doctor-patient relationship—clearly an important direct effect.

If you look in your Webster's dictionary, the primary definition of doctor is "teacher" not "healer." Teaching students from Liberty University Osteopathic School of Medicine, Lynchburg College's Physician Assistant, Physical Therapy, and Nurse Practitioner training programs efficiently extends a doctor's influence. This may take several forms from didactic lectures to mentoring in the clinic setting. When you're teaching, you're doctoring.

How important is a teacher? Several years ago, Randolph-Macon Woman's College hosted a retirement celebration for an outstanding economics professor. Charlie Gibson, CBS news anchor, was the featured speaker. Early in his career, he worked in Lynchburg and his wife taught at "Randy Mac." They maintained college contacts and were gracious enough to attend and give a presentation. Charlie started out asking a series of questions: "Who knows the CEO of (he then named each company, pausing for hands to be raised): IBM, GE, Hewlett Packard, GM?" A few hands went up as he mentioned each company. He followed with this question, "How many of you remember a teacher who had an important impact on your life?" All hands went up. That's how important a teacher is.

In a Master of Health Administration (MHA) course, I learned that the higher the level of community education, the healthier the community. This did not relate per se to community programs or seminars hosted by the hospital on specific diseases or health fairs. It meant the general public education level. A city or area with greater metrics of education such as reading level or high school graduation rate was healthier.

In addition to our excellent public school system, Lynchburg's general level of education is complemented by programs including after school tutoring programs, museums, and Amazement Square. Several physicians have served on the school board in the past. A unique effort spearheaded by Dr. Davis Von Oesen and his wife, Sally, is the E. C. Glass Foundation (see ECGlassFund.org for more information). It operates on the premise that quality teaching increases excellence in education. The foundation supports continued learning at all levels for teachers.

So, while the retired orthopedist is no longer performing joint replacement surgery, Dr. Von Oesen's involvement with the E. C. Glass Foundation improves the level of education and ergo makes a healthier community. He continues to impact the health of our community. If he's asked the question, "Didn't you used to be a doctor?" he can answer, "Yes, and I still am."

Most of my retired physician friends continue in activities such as the Free Clinic, missionary trips, teaching at all levels, and serving on health committees. We continue to be doctors.

# "IT'S SO NICE NOT TO SEE YOU"
## (Hypochondriacs Get Sick, Too; Murmurs)

She almost ran me down in the Boonsboro Shopping Center. Her Cutlass Cierra pulled up beside me, braked, and Evelyn's head popped out as she lowered the automatic window. "Dr. Jeff, it's so nice not to see you!"

Her comment was a compliment, not an insult. Six months earlier (May 1980), Evelyn came in my office with severe inflammatory arthritis in multiple joints. Some knuckles were red, swollen, tender and warm to touch. Her sedimentation rate was over 80 mm/hr (normal <10). She had hours of morning stiffness; her husband had to help dress her in the morning. Rheumatoid factor (RF) in her blood was elevated and I assumed she had a severe, fairly acute onset of rheumatoid arthritis. We added prednisone with anti-inflammatory meds, but she remained miserable with continued pain and disability.

She was followed by an excellent internal medicine group, and prior to her first office visit, I was forewarned by a phone call from her referring physician that Evelyn was a hypochondriac. In addition to a thoughtful note, her entire paper chart was sent over to my office for review. There were multiple ER notes for visits evaluating chest pain and fatigue. Heart attacks were ruled out. Occasionally, she was given a course of antibiotics for possible bronchitis, but usually the symptoms were attributed to stress and anxiety. As I reviewed the record, however, I noted a low grade fever recorded at several visits, and although seen in the ER by different on-call physicians from their practice, each doctor described a heart murmur that seemed to be worsening on subsequent visits. Hypochondriasis does not cause fever, heart murmur, elevated sedimentation rate, or inflammatory arthritis. Evelyn was sick.

A murmur is a sound produced by turbulence of irregular blood flow usually across an abnormal heart valve. As a rheumatologist, I never considered myself to be gifted in auscultation of the heart listening for murmurs. But even I heard the severe sound as blood rushed back into the heart across the aortic valve during diastole—when the heart relaxed after pumping blood out the aorta (systole). This was aortic insufficiency.

The rheumatoid factor (RF) test does not always indicate rheumatoid arthritis; it may be caused by infection in the heart (bacterial endocarditis). Could the arthritis be related to her heart murmur and possible infection? Blood cultures looking for active infection were negative on several occasions, and Evelyn's severe, painful arthritis persisted.

At this time in Lynchburg, we did not have invasive cardiology or infectious disease subspecialists. I arranged for an evaluation at Duke in infectious disease and cardiology. Dr. Dave Durack was an international expert on bacterial endocarditis. While they likewise could find no active infection, the heart was failing and aortic valve replacement was recommended.

Evelyn stayed in the hospital at Duke while cardiologists, cardiovascular surgeons, rheumatologists, and infectious disease specialists helped her prepare for surgery. I called Evelyn the night before surgery, expecting a state of anxiety. But she was calm and only concerned that she would receive a porcine valve (i.e. a valve made from pig valve material). I reassured her that the only problem would be at night, when all was quiet, she might hear an "oink" with each heartbeat. She was not amused.

Thankfully, the surgery went well. Dr. Durack thought that the removed valve probably had been damaged with an episode of endocarditis and perhaps the courses of antibiotics for bronchitis had partially treated and eventually eradicated the infection, but left an abnormal, leaking valve and progressive heart failure. Amazingly, over the next six weeks of rehabilitation, the arthritis resolved completely. The rheumatoid factor vanished and there were no signs of inflammation. Our Duke consultants felt that she had a reactive arthritis with the lab tests and clinical findings of inflammation resulting from the diseased heart valve.

Reactive arthritis is seen in several conditions (See…"Your Father Took Care of My Mother"). An infection normally stimulates the immune system. In some patients, after the infection is eradicated, the immune system continues to react against the patient's joints, causing a persistent inflammatory condition. Years ago, it was noted that some patients with severe gum disease and poor dentition had improvement in their arthritis when dental extractions and gum care eliminated the infectious element. In Evelyn's case, clearing infection with the episodic antibiotics for suspected bronchitis and replacing the damaged heart valve cured her arthritis.

Not only was it "nice not to see" me, but Evelyn added, "You put yourself out of business." Okay! That's the idea! My goal for all our patients was to control their arthritis, get it into remission, and perhaps cure them. If a curative therapy was available, I'd make sure they got the medicine, I would celebrate with them, hang up my shingle, and become the worst fishing guide on Smith Mountain Lake. An "Out of business—gone fishing" sign would hang on the office door.

Unfortunately, cures like this were rare. But Evelyn was a reminder that hypochondriacs also get sick. I remember a cartoon in one of our medical journals depicting the doctor in a graveyard looking at the inscription on his patient's headstone: "RIP" on top followed by "I told you I was sick" below it.

"Nice not to see me"? Her comment was a compliment, not an insult, and the feeling was mutual in the best sense.

## "I WANT ANOTHER ONE OF THOSE GOLD SHOTS"

## (Old Gold; Medicines—Risk, Reward, Remission)

Wow! You know you're dealing with an older rheumatologist when the topic is gold shots. Yes, real gold. No one could afford the treatment nowadays with the price of gold, but this was the first DMARD (Disease Modifying Anti-Rheumatic Drug) available, the first possible remittive agent for rheumatoid arthritis. And it was effective in many patients. It was given by injection starting with a 10 mg test dose, followed by a 25 mg shot and then weekly 50 mg doses.

But my patient S.C. (Susan), a fifty-seven-year-old white female, never got beyond the test dose of gold. The day after her 10 mg injection, she appeared with a reaction that looked like an acute attack of mononucleosis overnight. She was febrile, had swollen lymph nodes, elevated liver function tests, and high white blood cell count. She ached all over. This was a very rare reaction described in the medical literature, but I had never seen it before.

The gold treatment was stopped and the patient was started on a prednisone taper. Over the next two weeks, the rheumatoid arthritis was controlled beautifully with the prednisone, and the mono-like clinical and lab manifestations cleared. Susan and I awaited the expected return or flare of her arthritis after stopping the prednisone. But it never came. Instead, her rheumatoid arthritis went into complete remission for the next four years. My explanation for the response? The drug reaction, like most reactions, redirected the immune system. In this case, the gold "jolted" the immune system and stopped the autoimmune reaction against her joints.

179

Eventually, however, after four years the rheumatoid arthritis returned. That's when Susan said, "I want another one of those gold shots." I couldn't risk even another test dose of gold. "Are you kidding?" I exclaimed, "it could kill you and definitely would scare me to death. No way." I could understand her worry with the RA acting up again and the temptation of a four-year remission on no meds. It was worth the gamble to her. Fortunately, by now we had newer agents—specifically methotrexate, which controlled her arthritis.

The most common side effect of gold therapy was a skin rash. Diffuse, itchy, red with flat and raised areas (maculopapular) developed usually early in the course of the disease. Like most drug reactions, it meant the patient's immune system was irritated. Interestingly, we had found that patients who had gold skin reactions usually responded well as far as controlling the arthritis. After stopping the medicine, and allowing the rash to clear, the physician could often restart the gold therapy at a lower dose and maintain control of the illness without a recurrence of the rash. The lower dose of gold seemed to tweak the immune system enough to suppress the autoimmune process causing the RA, but not so much that an allergic drug reaction rash developed. It always reminded me of the ad on TV—"It's not nice to fool Mother Nature!" Don't push the immune system too far.

Methotrexate became the go-to initial DMARD. It could be given weekly by mouth rather than by injection, and while toxicity affecting the bone marrow causing low white count, anemia, and low platelets was similar to gold, methotrexate rarely caused any kidney toxicity, which could be a significant problem with gold therapy. The trade-off was more frequent testing to monitor for potential liver side effects (See… "I'm Not Taking That Damned Cancer Medicine").

Many of the DMARD medicines tread a fine line between controlling the immune system providing arthritis relief and aggravating an immune over-reaction provoking autoimmune disorders of their own. Penicillamine, for example, was an effective medicine for RA, but could cause autoimmune disorders including lupus, pemphigus, and myasthenia gravis in some patients. Its use demonstrates the constant problem of finding a balance between control of disease (reward) and adverse reactions to medications (risk).

While gold and penicillamine are rarely used now, the new biologic agents (such as Remicade, Enbrel, and Humira) continue the risk vs. reward conundrum. A one-minute TV commercial includes a fifteen second testimonial of miraculous effectiveness with forty-five seconds of caveats. The reward of great arthritis control is contrasted with the risk of fatal infection, cancers, or brain disease. Like our earlier agents, the biologics may be associated with the development of autoantibodies and features of diseases like drug-induced lupus. There are different classes of these agents acting against specific modulators of inflammation and joint destruction. Each may have unique side effects that may not be fully appreciated until their use is monitored over time.

If a patient failed treatment with the DMARDs (Disease Modifying Anti-rheumatic Drugs like methotrexate) and had a striking response to one of the biologic agents, reluctance to stop the medicine due to a side effect, with the risk of recurrent arthritis, is understandable. A prolonged remission off all meds, like Susan experienced after stopping gold, would be extremely rare.

If the RA remained active, I might try a different class of biologic agents, but I would avoid the old medicine even if the patient, like Susan, said, "I want another one of those" shots. The lesson Susan taught me, I refer to as the Golden Rule of Rheumatology—or an "Old Gold" Standard, still applicable to the new biologic agents. Another shot? Sorry, it would still be too risky for the patient and scary for this doctor.

# "...WITH A REACTION TO ONE OF YOUR MEDICINES"

## (Lynchburg Patients, Friends, and Neighbors)

Talk about guilt by association. A call from the Emergency Room physician came in the middle of morning office appointments, June 25,1990. "There's a patient here with a reaction to one of your medicines." M. B. was a forty-one-year-old white male working in Lynchburg on temporary assignment by his company. Fever and flu-like symptoms prompted the ER visit. He had long-standing severe, deforming rheumatoid arthritis and his lab studies showed a low WBC (white blood count), low platelet count, and elevated LFTs (liver function tests). The symptoms and lab tests could certainly be signs of toxicity from frequently used rheumatoid arthritis medicines like methotrexate or even gold shots. But he wasn't taking any of those meds, and I had never seen this patient.

Still, the combination of rheumatoid arthritis and abnormal lab tests was enough to merit referral to the rheumatologist. M. B. was very ill with a presumed infection perhaps on top of an impaired immune system sometimes related to Felty's Syndrome as part of long standing RA (See..."I Can't Believe You're Going Into Rheumatology"). But the problem was not his RA or one of "my" (the rheumatologist's) meds. M. B. had a rare blood condition (hematophagic histiocytosis), probably caused by a viral infection. In spite of excellent ICU (intensive care unit) nursing, consultations by infectious disease, hematology, and nephrology physicians, antibiotics, and extensive supportive care, the blood disorder could not be controlled, and M. B. died July 3, 1990.

Several years later, I was called by the Virginia Baptist ICU secretary. The primary physician wanted me to see his patient,

182

Betty Pearson, who was hospitalized "with a reaction to one of your medicines." Unlike M. B., this sixty-eight-year-old white female was my rheumatology patient treated with methotrexate for an inflammatory arthritis. Abnormal labs included a low WBC and abnormal LFTs. These were parameters we followed routinely monitoring for possible toxicity to methotrexate, and a review of office records revealed no previous abnormal lab tests.

Was something else going on? Betty was not only a patient, but a personal friend who lived in the same neighborhood around Bedford Hills Elementary School. She had served as the secretary of the Lynchburg Academy of Medicine for several years including my year as Academy president. She was really an executive director, an invaluable resource for the entire medical community. Now retired, she maintained a regular morning brisk walk routine while her husband, Bob, walked the dog and retrieved the morning paper. I saw them both frequently as I drove to work along Burnt Bridge Road.

In the ICU, Betty was febrile and slightly disoriented, a far cry from the healthy walker I knew. Since recent routine lab monitoring tests had been normal, a drug reaction to methotrexate seemed unlikely, and considering the combination of outdoor and canine exposure, I ordered blood tests for tick borne diseases. The tests revealed that Betty had Lyme disease and ehrlichiosis, two tick related diseases—not a reaction to her arthritis meds.

Years later, during my last few months in practice, Bob had a scheduled office visit to follow his osteoarthritis. Progressive weakness and fatigue were limiting the usual morning routine of walking the dog and retrieving his newspaper. While he attributed this to age, the change in six months was striking and worrisome. These symptoms and worsening joint pains in the setting of possible tick exposure gratis the dog, suggested a tick-related problem in spite of no known bite. The Lyme test was positive and this was the one case of Lyme disease I diagnosed in my last fifteen months of practice, while finding 147 patients

(+) for alpha gal tick disease (See..."My Doctor Thinks I Have Lupus").

As physicians, we always consider medicine reactions in our differential diagnosis as we try to determine the cause of our patient's symptoms. But sometimes, it's not a problem with their meds. Then other factors may be important in providing clues to a diagnosis. Continuity of care (knowing Betty's prior labs and Bob's prior level of activity) as well as familiarity with physical surroundings and habits of people (walking dogs in an area with abundant deer and tick population), may all help direct our tests and treatment.

This is part of the uniqueness of Lynchburg explained to me by Dr. George Craddock years ago. Our patients are our neighbors and friends. As a physician, you not only care for them (provide medical services), you care about them (the intangibles of the art of medicine). The result is special medical care exemplified by the late Dr. Craddock.

## "I WOULD HAVE BEEN DISMISSED FROM THE PRACTICE"
## (Socialized Medicine)

Ian was a sixty-five-year-old Scot. Although he had been in Lynchburg over ten years working as an engineer and was a naturalized U.S. citizen, he reminded me of my late mother-in-law who was a WWII war bride from Scotland; once a Scot, always a Scot. He had long-standing, severe rheumatoid arthritis, but now had a new complaint. He was bothered by mild swelling in his lower legs. The most common cause would be dependent edema with excess fluid settling in the legs during the day. Restricting salt in the diet and a mild fluid pill should take care of it.

When the swelling did not improve by the time of his two-week follow-up visit, Ian questioned my diagnostic and treatment approach. "Why didn't you check my kidney function? Couldn't the naproxen medicine you put me on cause kidney damage and swelling?" It was more of a challenge than an innocent inquiry. I could only reply, "You're right, Ian. Although dependent edema would be much more common, we need to check the kidneys and stop the naproxen, which could cause swelling and renal problems."

Indeed, the urinalysis showed abnormal loss of protein and red blood cells in the urine. Lab studies showed mildly abnormal kidney function. His past medical history from Scotland days included a chronic problem of hematuria (blood in the urine) and I referred him to the kidney specialist. He was diagnosed with an unusual ailment—IgA nephropathy. The swelling was a sign that the condition was worsening, and the nephrologist explained that, not only was it not related to the naproxen, but the trial of a mild diuretic fluid pill was appropriate.

By the time of his next office visit, the nephrologist's re-assurance made Ian more contented with his rheumatology care. Somewhat chagrined, he said, "Do you know what would have happened to me in Scotland if I questioned the doctor? I would have been dismissed from the practice." Convenient, I thought, but not honest. During the time he was under social-ized medicine in Scotland, all the care was directed through the local primary care doctor. Financial constraints and a shortage of subspecialists in rheumatology and nephrology would have complicated and delayed further evaluation or care.

The only knowledge I had about the British health care system came from two sources. Dr. Robert Sydnor, one of our finest orthopedic surgeons, spent some time in England as a medical student. He recalled having a patient's visit in the office consultation room interrupted at tea time. First things first, Old Chap. The patient seemed to understand and accept this.

More alarming was the story of a patient seen with a dis-secting abdominal aortic aneurysm—basically like a blow-out ready to occur on a tire, but in this case involving the major blood vessel coming out of the heart—clearly a life threatening emergency. Bob called the operating room to prepare for sur-gery as quickly as possible. The operating room nurse, however, called the attending physician. This Yank medical student didn't understand how the system worked. There was no emergency surgery. The patient would be monitored with meds to lower blood pressure and surgery would be scheduled the next day electively, a risky delay. Even over forty years ago when this occurred, it was not the standard of care in the United States.

The other source of information that impressed me came through what we physicians called "throw away journals,"— free publications with lots of pharmaceutical ads and excellent summary articles as well. *Hospital Practice* and *Hospital Medi-cine* were two of my favorite publications full of pictures and algorithms.

In the mid-1980s, there was debate regarding patients with unstable angina—a heart condition worrisome for an im-pending heart attack. Nationally, the majority of our colleagues favored a more aggressive approach. Perform cardiac catheter-ization as soon as possible, define the status of the coronary arteries and proceed with coronary artery bypass grafts as in-dicated (this was before stents were available). The alternative was medical therapy.

As I reviewed an algorithm for unstable angina in an is-sue of *Hospital Practice,* I noted the usual two major divisions branching out to cardiac cath and surgery versus medicines only. I was surprised that cardiac catheterization was not offered to all the patients, with medicine treatment alone for patients whose caths showed changes that would not be amenable to bypass surgery. Although I was only forty years old at the time, I was surprised as I traced the paths to the point where they divided. The determinant for aggressive cath and surgery treat-ment or conservative medical therapy was age. Anyone over fifty-five years of age was assigned to medical therapy alone; under fifty-five you qualified for catheterization and surgery.

Where did this come from? It clearly was not the standard of care in our country. The authors were physicians at Guy's Hospital in London. Any physician has to be impressed with the difference between chronologic and physiologic age. One eighty-year-old may be physiologically younger than a fifty-year-old obese patient who is a chain smoker. An arbitrary de-termination of fifty-five years or any chronologic age is ridicu-lous, and I hope has changed since then.

But shortly after Ian's visit, he brought me a copy of an article from the *London Times.* A young lady in the midst of her first pregnancy had so many questions regarding the pri-mary care physician's therapy that he dismissed her from his practice—and he dismissed her husband as well. Guilt by as-sociation or guilt by conception? Maybe Ian was feeling grate-ful he had not been dismissed, and hopefully these features of socialized medicine will never be part of our country's quest for affordable care.

# "BUT IT'S AS BAD AS CANCER, ISN'T IT?"
## (Scleroderma)

I had to answer, "Yes, it's as bad as cancer."

M. C. was a sixty-seven-year-old African American female with a ten-year history of scleroderma. Her primary doctor hospitalized her at VBH (Virginia Baptist Hospital) to evaluate chest pain with irregular heartbeats (palpitations), and he requested a rheumatology consultation. She had been followed at the University of Virginia Rheumatology Clinic, and although I had never seen her before, her story was not unusual for scleroderma.

More than ten years ago, she noted Raynaud's phenomenon affecting her fingers. With cold exposure, the fingers would blanch and begin the classic progression of white to blue to red color changes. Gradually, the skin on her fingers began to tighten and thicken as a sign of "scleroderma"—"hard skin." Sores with calcium deposits (calcinosis) developed and red spots (telangiectasias) appeared on her skin. In spite of excellent care at the medical center, the patient developed breathing problems requiring twenty-four hour a day oxygen therapy. Shortness of breath was exacerbated by the least exertion. Rising from a seated position and walking a few steps exhausted M. C.

Her only question after I examined her was, "It's not cancer, is it?" I reassured her that there were no signs of cancer. However, over the next week, M. C. had three episodes of cardiac arrest. Code blue was called each time, and irregular heart rhythms were corrected, sometimes requiring electric shocks. Every day as I saw her on my hospital rounds, she repeated the same question. But after the third arrest, she changed her question, "It's not cancer, but it's as bad as cancer, isn't it?"

I had to answer, "Yes, it's as bad as cancer." M. C. died during that hospital admission from respiratory failure and cardiac arrest. It was 1983, and over the next thirty years of practice, scleroderma would continue to be a severe, devastating disease.

As a systemic disease, it had many different manifestations. Two patients, Marion Weaver and Laurie Babcock, developed the disease about the same time in the mid to late 1980s. I met with each patient and family members outlining the serious nature of scleroderma and the likelihood that it could be a fatal illness within five to ten years. Each patient initially presented with pain and mild swelling of the fingers as well as Raynaud's phenomenon, but over time their diseases took different courses.

Marion Weaver was fifty-eight years old and director of the Miller Home for Girls when first seen February 5, 1987. Over the years, sclerodactly—"hard" fingers with recurrent painful infections occurred, and pulmonary fibrosis developed in her lungs. She was treated with calcium channel blocker meds like Procardia to control the Raynaud's phenomenon. Low dose prednisone and penicillamine were used to slow down the fibrosing or scarring nature of scleroderma. The meds were of moderate benefit, and she was able to continue work and retire from her Miller Home director's duties in 1992. She and her husband, Bruce, remained active in many church and community affairs including Churches for Urban Ministry where my wife, Sandra, witnessed and shared their devotion to that organization. Over the next twenty-two years, Marion's main symptoms were due to progressively more painful, infected fingers with recurrent sores and gradual cardiovascular problems including postural hypotension.

Marion died August 27, 2014. Her obituary not only mentioned her church and work activities, but touched on the unique nature of Lynchburg medicine. After caring for her over three decades and appreciating the volunteer work with Sandra, Marion and Bruce were more like friends than patient and husband. One of my mentors in medicine, Eugene A. Stead, Jr., observed that over time as you cared for a patient, you did not see the disease in the patient, you saw the person in the disease.

How true. I was humbled by a note in the obituary: "She especially honored the life-saving care she received from Dr. Jeff Wilson, Rheumatologist, throughout her thirty-year battle with Scleroderma." It *was* a battle, and I was privileged to be part of it as her physician and friend.

Laurie Babcock and her family were likewise personal friends. Unfortunately, Laurie's illness quickly involved the lungs in a more severe manner with pulmonary hypertension and pulmonary fibrosis. Like several of my patients, she was followed every six months at the MUSC (Medical University of South Carolina) center in Charleston. Dr. Richard Silver and his colleagues had special expertise in scleroderma lung disease. Their recommended course of intravenous Cytoxan (cyclophosphamide), along with low dose prednisone stabilized the scleroderma for a while, but in 2004, shortness of breath became more severe as pulmonary function worsened. During this time, Laurie continued to work with Bobby at Babcock's Auto Service (usually assisted by their yellow lab), began a cookbook with friends (*Seasons To Taste*, Blackwell Press 2009), arranged a beautiful wedding for their daughter, Tucker, and maintained a strong faith (See..."One Of Your Patients Prayed For You Today").

When a repeat trial of intravenous Cytoxan and prednisone failed to improve or stabilize her pulmonary function, a lung transplant was suggested. By now, Laurie required continuous oxygen therapy and medical center input was sought at several centers including Johns Hopkins. Oxygen saturation, an indicator of lung function, is measured by a pulse oximeter and should run 96 to 100 percent. Gradually her resting oxygen saturation decreased into the 80 percent range, falling dangerously low with minimal exertion.

The Johns Hopkins Medical Center evaluation included bronchoalveolar lavage (washing the lungs out to detect any inflammatory cells that might suggest a beneficial treatment). This had to be scheduled December 14, 2004, as a single day, outpatient procedure because insurance would not pay for hospitalization in spite of Laurie's progressively fragile pulmonary status. The trip concluded with a harrowing drive home as oxygen saturation dropped, Laurie felt cold, and her extremities became cyanotic (discolored blue from lack of oxygen). Tony Piggott, a close friend, and sister, Meg Laughon, accompanied Laurie. They took turns massaging Laurie's arms and hands to improve the circulation and warm her all the way home. Meg remembers changing oxygen canisters more frequently than usual. "Laurie was sucking up the oxygen as fast as she could." The procedure and trip left her tired, weak, with severe oxygen deficiency. Imagine the fear and anxiety Tony and Meg experienced driving through that dark, cold wintry night with their friend and sister becoming progressively short of breath.

Laurie was not a lung transplant candidate due to gastrointestinal reflux. The gradual progression of her disease was causing a slow suffocation from lack of oxygen. At one point, she was notified by her insurance company that she had used up her quota of oxygen! It seemed that as she got sicker, support from her health insurance lessened, but the support of friends and family increased.

Laurie wrote a letter to the editor of the *News & Advance* the week before she died titled "When health insurance becomes unaffordable" outlining the problem of the medical industrial complex and the failed promise of a PHO (Physician Hospital Organization) for its community.

## When Health Insurance Becomes Unaffordable

### By Laurie Babcock

Life holds no guarantees and we accept this premise in exchange for a certain degree of fairness and justice in the circumstances that come our way. We work hard to provide for our family and employees, protecting them from potential devastation or catastrophic events. In this country we believe in a free enterprise that provides insurance against such times. We understand that we may not always be able to absorb such debilitating costs, so we look to an industry that can protect us from financial ruin. This system is based on a trust between the provider and the members—an assurance that life will continue even in these most difficult times.

The Piedmont Community Health Plan Web site states that it is an insurance company which is "owned and operated by people you know and trust—more than 250 local physicians and Centra Health, our local hospital system—a program designed by the local medical community which promotes the concept that your physician will manage your care." This insurance plan seemed ideal. Certainly, they would know the difficulties and hardships in times of a serious disease or illness.

Three years ago my husband and I decided to move his automobile repair shop's group health plan to PCHP. The concept was one that we approved: a policy that was managed by people we know and a comprehensive plan that was beneficial to our employees. We disclosed at this time a chronic autoimmune disease that I had been battling for 10 years. After discussing this with PCHP, we signed a contract that we believed was fair.

Last winter, this disease took a turn for the worse and I developed a severe interstitial lung disease. Within three months my lungs were operating at 20 percent, and I was on 24-hour continuous oxygen. I was put on a lung transplant list as the only option of saving me from this life-threatening situation. PCHP had agreed to pay for this procedure, but in November when our company contract with them came up for renewal, we were devastated. Our premium had been raised by 247 percent—from an annual cost of $22,000 to more than $76,000. The increase was one no small business could absorb. Our choices were few: we could drop our company health plan or we could accept whatever price the insurance market dictated. For me, there were no options.

Here in Central Virginia we are blessed with many fine companies that provide our citizens with the best possible services. Unfortunately, sometimes business decisions dictate consequences that are not beneficial to our community.

Centra Health, one of two majority shareholders in PCHP, is in the midst of a major capital campaign. It is asking the people of this area to support a construction project that will provide the latest in medical technology and treatments. In my opinion, as part of the decision-making process of PCHP, the hospital is also responsible for denying affordable access to the state of the art facility. Without health insurance, who can afford to pay for these services? I know that neither our company nor our employees can.

We expect our community businesses to deal with us in a fair and just manner. This is not something we should be willing to sacrifice for the sake of a "sound business decision" that benefits the stockholders over the people who entrust their health and lives to them. It is a shame that Piedmont Community Health Plan has demonstrated that it is willing to make just such a sacrifice.

Addendum: PCHP is now totally owned and operated by Centra. It is no longer a PHO (Physician Hospital Organization).

On the Sunday prior to Laurie's final hospitalization, I was called to her home. The first floor looked like a hospital room with bed, oxygen tank, ice chips, and blankets. Laurie had a coterie of wonderful friends including Kitty Bass, Gale Mudrick, Betty Jo Hamner, Melissa Johnson, Cindy Warren, Becky O'Brian, and Rhonda Clower. I witnessed Laurie's friends caring for her. Massage, adjust pillows, fix food, assist with the oxygen—anything to comfort and support her was provided in an atmosphere of love and concern.

After examining her, I felt there might be an element of treatable infection or inflammation that could improve her shortness of breath, but it would be handled best in the hospital. Although Laurie's physical condition was weakened, her spirit and will remained strong. While she would consider hospital treatment, the final decision depended on which physician was taking calls for pulmonary medicine. When she found out it was Dr. Steve Johnson, she agreed to go. Unfortunately, Laurie died during that hospitalization on February 7, 2005. I was honored to be her physician, friend, and pallbearer.

Sir William Osler, one of the godfathers of clinical medicine, said that the appropriate thing for the doctor to do when the arthritis patient came in the front door was to go out the back door. This was based on the limited treatment modalities available for arthritis in the early 1900s. One of my clinical instructors during rheumatology training suggested that, in this time of modern medicine, the same advice might apply for the scleroderma patient. While some aspects of the disease may be "as bad as cancer" when the physician and patient find themselves frustrated by ineffective therapies, the experience with all my scleroderma patients has allowed me to witness great courage and faith. Avoiding them, or "going out the back door," would have been as great a loss for me as for the patient because in each case, as Dr. Stead suggested, I did not find a disease in a patient. Instead, I witnessed a remarkable person in the disease.

# ABOUT THE AUTHOR

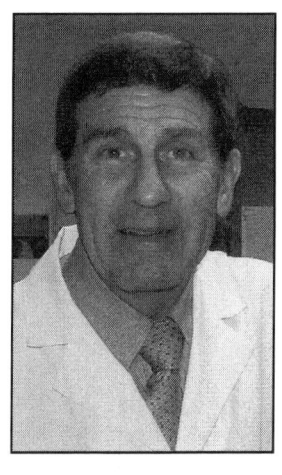

Dr. Wilson was born in Charleston, West Virginia, but lived in Connecticut, Kentucky, Florida, and Pennsylvania while growing up. He is Duke inbred, receiving a BS in Zoology (1968) and his M.D. in 1972. He continued postgraduate medical training at Duke including internship, internal medicine residency, and rheumatology fellowship from 1972 till 1979. This was interrupted by two years of active duty Navy service (1974-1976).

He and his wife, Sandra, have been married since June 20, 1969. They have two children, Elizabeth and Melissa, and three grandchildren. The longest he has lived in any one place has been Lynchburg where he practiced rheumatology from July 7, 1979, until December 15, 2014.

He previously wrote *"Hello, Friend" Dr. George B. Craddock Stories* (Warwick House Publishing, 1989) and has authored articles in medical journals and a chapter "Vitamin D and Sjögren's Syndrome" in *The Sjögren's Book* (Oxford University Press, 2012).

He served as President of the Lynchburg Academy of Medicine, 6th District Councilor to the Medical Society of Virginia, and was the tenth recipient of the William Barney Award in 2007. He and Sandra reside in Lynchburg.

Dr. Wilson may be contacted at 434-444-1729 or by email at Wilson1821@Comcast.net.